The Natural
Makeover Diet

The Natural Makeover Diet

A 4-STEP PROGRAM TO LOOKING
AND FEELING YOUR BEST FROM
THE INSIDE OUT

DR. JOEY SHULMAN

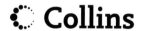

HarperCollins books may be purchased for educational, business, or sales
promotional use through our Special Markets Department.

HarperCollins Publishers Ltd
2 Bloor Street East, 20th Floor
Toronto, Ontario, Canada
M4W 1A8

www.harpercollins.ca

Library and Archives Canada Cataloguing in Publication
information is available upon request.

ISBN 978-1-44342-798-2

Printed and bound in the United States of America
RRD 9 8 7 6 5 4 3 2 1

For my family, with love—Randy, Jonah and Faith

contents

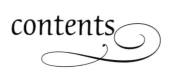

acknowledgments

I am thrilled to have the opportunity to re-release *The Natural Makeover Diet*.

Since first writing this book, I have had the great blessing of working with thousands of men and women, helping them to achieve their goal weight and feel and look their very best by following the principles outlined in these pages. For those who have taken the leap to improve their health and have allowed me to be their "coach" along the way, I thank you. Your health transformations are truly an inspiration to me and others. I must also thank my amazing team at the Shulman Weight Loss Clinics. Their devotion to health and our clients continues to change lives daily.

With any project I do, it is always my family's love and support that is the backbone. Mom, Dad, Laina and Danny—you are always there to cheer me on and I love you all so much. Lain ... for every phone call and every email—what I know for sure is that I could not do it without you. To my kids—Jonah and Faith—I am truly blessed to be your mom. It is my greatest joy, and I adore both of you.

Finally, to my husband—and the love of my life—Randy: for your patience with my worrying ways (sorry ... working on it!), your love and unrelenting support—I thank you. You are my *besheret* and we are still having the best good time. Truly, madly and deeply.

With the re-release of *The Natural Makeover Diet*, you will discover new recipes, updated research and information and tips that will help you reach your ultimate health goals and look and feel your very best ... naturally.

Wishing you best health on this journey,

Dr. Joey Shulman DC, RNCP

introduction

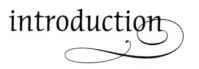

"You can't look good if you don't feel good!"
—Anonymous

Your face does not lie. You can determine the state of health a woman is in simply by looking at her skin, hair and nails. If you are sick or run down on the inside, it always shows on the outside in myriad ways such as bags under the eyes, dry skin, brittle nails, premature wrinkling, excess weight or difficulty losing weight. Yet, the norm in today's society is to cover up the signs of poor health instead of addressing them. Women of all ages are turning to external quick fixes such as makeup, tanning beds and even risky surgical procedures in the name of beauty. In truth, the key to looking your best throughout your life is to deal with your inside health first. Once you start taking care of your internal health, your natural beauty will shine through each and every time in the form of wrinkle-free skin and a radiant complexion, sparkling eyes, strong nails, shiny hair and a natural shift towards a healthy and normal body weight. For women searching to enhance their looks, the process of "finding their natural beauty" begins with nutritious food, proper exercise, the right minerals, vitamins and fats and a proper cleanse. I assure you, this is by far the most effective and long-lasting makeover available.

When first discussing the potential of this book with my publisher, I became very excited about the idea of offering this information to women of all ages. As a former model, I witnessed the toll that smoking, a poor diet and stress eventually took on many beautiful women at a very young age. Women in their 20s started to look older than they should, due to the acceleration of certain physiological processes, which I will outline in chapter 2. In my current career as a practicing health care professional dedicated to holistic and natural approaches to women's health, I have had the opportunity to combine my knowledge of integrative (holistic) health care with my passion for helping women achieve external beauty—to look and feel their best. The results are by far the most powerful beauty and health changes I have had the pleasure of witnessing.

Under the Knife

When examining the statistics of cosmetic surgery, I discovered that 90 percent of all cosmetic surgical procedures are performed on women. While it is no secret that every woman wants to look good, this begs the question: Is turning to a knife, chemical peel or expensive lotion really the answer? While I am an advocate of taking the steps to do what makes you feel good, I am concerned that as a society, we are becoming obsessed with external, often risky and unnecessary measures in the name of beauty. This book is by no means intended as a critique and "bashing" of cosmetic procedures; it is rather a guide to show women how to achieve their optimal body weight, beautiful skin and healthy glow with natural, non-invasive approaches.

The focus on external beauty and the temptation to hang on to youth is deeply ingrained in our society. This is evident in the enormous surge in reality television shows doing intense "before and after" shots of women and men feeling bothered by anything from their teeth, hair and body weight to their nose and breasts. From tummy tucks and Botox parties to liposuction and buttock lifts, high-risk and expensive procedures to achieve a picture-perfect look are definitely taking hold. Sounds crazy, doesn't it? Women undergo high-risk surgical procedures and injections with long-term potential health consequences—all in the name of appearances! Now, I am of course not suggesting that my approach to beauty can create the same results as a nose job or getting your teeth done. However, in terms of achieving optimal energy, beautiful skin, your ideal body weight and that unmistakable "glow," the results from natural approaches win hands down.

The popularity of cosmetic surgical approaches is evident by the millions of dollars spent on procedures each and every year. In 2004, the number of cosmetic plastic surgery procedures increased 5 percent with more than 9.2 million procedures performed. To put this into perspective, according to the American Society of Plastic Surgeons (ASPS), this growth rate is steady with that of the U.S. economy!

The top five cosmetic procedures performed in 2012 were nose reshaping (243,000), liposuction (202,000), breast augmentation (286,000), eyelid surgery (204,000) and facelift (126,000). Consider the following:

- Americans spent $10.4 billion on cosmetic surgery in 2011.
- In 2011, breast implants were still number one, with 307,180 surgeries.

- Americans forked over more than $38 million on chin jobs last year, having one every 25 minutes. This procedure costs an average of $1,851.

- In 2012, plastic surgeons were the seventh-highest ranked specialists, with a mean income of $317,000. Topping the list were orthopedists, cardiologists, radiologists, gastroenterologists and urologists.

Looking Good

"You look marvelous!"

—Billy Crystal, comedian

Our society places great value on outer beauty. We feel better about ourselves if we look (or think we look) better. This notion was evidenced by a greeting card that I recently saw. The cover read: "Good clothes open all doors!" On a certain level, there is a deeper truth to this statement. Trust me, I am all for looking good and feeling your best. We all walk into a room with a little more confidence and pep in our step if we think we have it "going on." Feeling good about the way your skin, hair and nails look, the way your body appears and how you are dressed tends to change the way you deal with your family, business associates and even yourself in quiet moments. However, my belief supported by my observations in practice is that the most beautiful you is best revealed by taking natural steps, not surgical ones. When inner health is achieved, your deepest level of beauty shines through. There is a certain sparkle or glow that is achieved when you follow the four steps outlined in this book which include 1) cleanse, 2) nourish, 3) moisturize and 4) maintenance.

Broccoli or Botox?

In the midst of the surge in plastic surgery procedures, there is another trend taking place. People are spending dramatically more of their hard-earned dollars on natural health and preventative medicine. Slowly but surely, the message is getting out that wholesome eating, regular exercise and proper supplementing with minerals, vitamins and essential fats is the most effective way to prevent disease, prolong and optimize life and maintain and enhance your looks. There is no pill, potion or lotion that comes even close to achieving the results of proper nutrition.

As with cosmetic surgery, women are also the leading consumers in natural health products. Women are motivated and eager to gather all the information they can about everything from food safety to supplementing properly in order to shop better, to keep their families healthier and to maintain and preserve their health, beauty and quality of life. According to data from the 1998/99 National Population Health Survey (NPHS):

- Nutrition tends to be more important to women than men.
- Women are more likely to use vitamins regularly.
- Women are more likely than men to consider overall health, weight and specific diseases when choosing food.
- 80 percent of women are concerned about maintaining or improving health through food choices, compared with 63 percent of men.
- 59 percent of women consider their weight when selecting foods, whereas just 41 percent of men do.

- About 48 percent of women consider the relationship between food and heart disease, compared with 38 percent of men.

The Misnomer of Anti-Aging

When searching the market for natural beauty options, consumers will likely find many programs and books with the term "anti-aging" in the title. In reality, this term is misleading. Although you may not want to hear this, *the aging process cannot and should not be stopped!* Aging is a natural occurrence that helps the body to evolve from one fundamental stage to another. Instead of focusing on an unachievable state of anti-aging, it is far wiser and effective to embrace a process that allows you to age well with a natural mind and body approach. By working with, not against, the aging process, you can look and feel 10 to 20 years younger when you are in your 50s, 60s and 70s! The premise of this book is based on the following principle: *In order to reveal the most beautiful you at any age, changes must be made from the inside out.* Whether you have dark circles under your eyes, wrinkles or acne, the key to a successful and natural makeover begins by addressing the aging accelerators within the body. Once these are addressed, health changes such as sparkling eyes, glowing skin and a svelte body will be the ultimate pay-off.

The Beauty Robbers

After years of clinical experience, I have had the opportunity to clearly map and identify the top three "beauty robbers." Beauty robbers can be defined as physiological processes that speed up the aging process in an unnatural and accelerated fashion. When this occurs, women in their 20s, 30s or 40s appear and feel older than their actual biological age. However, with the proper information and nutritional and lifestyle approach, these processes can be halted and even reversed in a very short time. Because of our body's forgiving nature and extraordinary healing abilities, once given the proper nourishment, supplements and hydration, you will see changes in just one week. When you start implementing the 4-step program outlined in *The Natural Makeover Diet*, your body will shift back to its rightful place of optimal health and wellness. Within the first week of implementing the 4-step program, you will begin to notice subtle changes such as your skin clearing, pounds coming off and an increase in energy. Within two to four weeks, the changes will become more dramatic and long lasting.

This book provides you with a detailed explanation of the top three beauty robbers which are:

1. Faulty digestion
2. Chronic inflammation
3. Free radical damage

By following the 4-step beauty and health program outlined in chapters 3–6, you will turn beauty robbers into beauty enhancers. In other words, the physiological processes that were once making you look and feel older than you are will now work for you.

Starting the Program

As mentioned above, the Natural Makeover Diet involves four steps to looking and feeling your best. They are:

1. Cleanse (for five days)

2. Nourish

3. Moisturize

4. Maintenance

I recommend first reading the entire book to gain as much knowledge as you can before starting the program. It is very important for everyone to have an understanding of how their body works and the proper natural steps necessary to heal and maintain optimal health. In my practice, I have found that those who understand the *why* behind what they are doing tend to heal faster and respond better. This is due to the powerful connection between the mind and the body. However, I understand that some of you are eager to start the processes immediately so you can begin feeling and living the results. If this is the case, simply flip to the back of chapters 3–6 for summary pages of how to begin. That way, you can read the additional information at your leisure. The first step of the program includes a five-day cleansing period. Five days is the perfect amount of time to cleanse. I recommend doing the five-day cleanse from a Monday to a Friday as weekends are often the time when people "fall off the health wagon." Following those initial five days, steps 2, 3 and 4 of the program are all followed at the same time.

In chapters 7 and 8, you will find additional information on the top health optimizers and answers to frequently asked questions such as what is a safe sugar substitute, is soy safe to eat and is butter really better than margarine? At the back of the book you will also find must-have recipes for quick, easy and delicious options to tempt your palate.

I sincerely believe that health and wellness is every person's birthright, not a privilege. I applaud you for taking this journey towards reclaiming and maximizing your own inner health and wellness. I am excited to hear about your beauty results! Please feel free to let me know how the "new you" looks and feels at www.drjoey.com. I always welcome natural "before" and "after" pictures!

Wishing you best health and happiness,
Dr. Joey Shulman DC, RNCP

chapter

YOUR HEALTH STATUS

"The best part of beauty is that which no picture can express."

—SIR FRANCIS BACON

*Y*our body, in its innate wisdom, has several checks and balance systems that take place on a minute-by-minute basis, ensuring that all systems are a "go" and everything is running as smoothly as possible. From neurotransmitters (brain chemicals) firing in your brain to mucous secretions taking place in the small intestine to white blood cells fighting off infection—the symphony of your body's continual operating and healing process is nothing short of miraculous. However, like most things in life, your body can only undergo a certain amount of abuse before the smooth running of this fine-tuned engine runs up against interference. Unfortunately, the elements that cause the slow (or sometimes fast, depending on your genetic makeup) deterioration of your health and beauty have become commonplace in the Western world. Our health and wellness takes continual abuse from practices such as eating trans fats, fast foods, refined sugars and flours, consuming too little essential fats, fruits and vegetables, smoking, stress, lack of exercise and dehydration.

I'm Sorry, Body!

Luckily for all of us, our bodies have an incredibly forgiving nature. Even after years of abuse, if given the proper conditions, the body forgives the sins of the past and has the incredible capacity to heal itself, halt disease and revert to its rightful state of health and wellness. So, you may ask, "How does this relate to outer beauty and the way I look?" I assure you, in order for you to look your best, you must deal with the "inside factor" first. Once you deal with your inside factor, the changes you will notice will be different than those achieved by surgical procedures, tanning beds or cosmetic applications. The natural glow and sparkle achieved by following the 4-step program results in a noticeable radiance that only comes from reaching a state of internal wellness. In addition, you will avoid risky side effects that commonly accompany surgery and medication such as infection and lengthy healing time. The program is natural, easy to apply to your lifestyle, offers delicious food choices and provides you with the tools to achieve all of your health and beauty goals.

Your Genes

When I was studying anatomy, each student was assigned to a cadaver for dissection and learning purposes. In the anatomy lab I was witness to the internal makeup of the human body; I was astonished at how similar each and every human being was. It was fascinating to me that we all, for the most part, have the same layout of veins, arteries and nerves. From the intricate road map of our arterial system to the muscles in our legs—it is all virtually the same!

As I entered practice and started to see patients, it became obvious to me that although our internal systems may look virtually identical on the inside, each individual is biochemically different and responds in various ways to external factors that affect our health. This is why two individuals can be exposed to the flu virus and Person A will develop the flu and Person B will not. Another example of this is the lucky individual who can eat an abundant amount of fast food and refined sugars and still maintain a lean body weight (trust me, they are a rare breed!), whereas someone else will become obese and develop Type II diabetes by eating the same diet. In other words, we all have a different genetic coding that determines our resiliency to disease and our current state of health. This phenomenon is what I refer to as "the George Burns principle of health." George Burns, one of the funniest entertainers of the twentieth century, always had a cigar in hand, drank alcohol and surely ate plenty of inflammatory foods. Mr. Burns, holding his ever-present cigar, was asked what his doctor thought about his smoking. Mr. Burns retorted, "My doctor is dead!"

Even by doing all of the wrong things healthwise, George lived to the ripe old age of 100 in a state of good health and alertness. On the flipside, George was also very social, loved people and had a wonderful marriage which certainly plays a significant role in overall health. There are many people who do not have the same resiliency that George's system did, and given the same conditions would develop heart disease or cancer and would perhaps even succumb to a disease at a much earlier age. Although we may all look the same on the inside, we each respond very differently to our surroundings, our food, our thoughts and our activity level.

The Puzzle Pieces of Health

> "Some people think that doctors and nurses can put scrambled eggs back into the shell."
> —Unknown

The body is made of various systems such as the cardiovascular, immune, nervous and digestive systems. Although these systems are talked about as separate entities, they are not. Like various instruments coming together to form a beautiful piece of music, all systems in the body flow together and communicate to ensure optimal health. This is a new concept for many to understand because the current medical model is designed on the basis of the body comprising separate systems. For example, if you have a digestive system problem such as Crohn's disease, you visit a gastroenterologist. For a heart condition, you see a cardiologist. For severe pains in your knees, you probably see an orthopedic surgeon. Of course, there is a time and a place for medication and surgery such as emergency situations, pain relief or for disease processes that have gone too far. Yet, I believe that integrative medicine that emphasizes a holistic approach and prevention through diet, exercise and lifestyle management offers the key to achieving internal health and external beauty. When used as a preventative tool or as a strategy to reverse disease processes, natural medicine is an equally powerful "brother" to the conventional medical model.

While most people are familiar with the benefit of holistic approaches to healthcare, curiously, many are not putting these fundamentals of wellness into action in their own lives. People are not putting together the puzzle pieces of their own current state of health. For example, aspects such as food, mood, disease and exercise are all interrelated. I am routinely shocked by overweight patients who seem genuinely surprised that they have developed other ailments such as high blood pressure, Type II diabetes, depression and lower back pain. Instead of seeing the connection, they react as if they have been unlucky to "get" so many illnesses and disease processes. In truth, all their health concerns stem from the same cause. The core problem is faulty nutrition, which causes excess weight, stress on the heart (high blood pressure), stress on the joints (lower back pain) and fluctuations in blood sugar and insulin control (Type II diabetes).

Although doctors attempt to get to the bottom of specific health problems, their method of training often just masks the symptom with medication rather than taking care of the problem. If you have reflux disease, an antacid or an HCI inhibitor drug is recommended. Do you have high blood pressure? A diuretic pill is often prescribed. Are you suffering from depression? How about an anti-depressant? Instead of using symptoms as a clue to discover the predisposing factor that is ailing the body, doctors often think that the disease or disorder is cured if the symptom is silenced. The growing trend of treating the symptom and not going after the source is evidenced by the billions of dollars we spend yearly on medications. The following chart highlights the top 10 most popular drugs prescribed in 2010.

Table 1.1: The Top 10 Most Popular Drugs Prescribed in 2010

Drug	Action	US billions spent
Lipitor	Cholesterol-lowering statin	$7.2
Nexium	Antacid	$6.3
Plavix	Blood thinner	$6.1
Advair Diskus	Asthma inhaler	$4.7
Abilify	Antipsychotic	$4.6
Seroquel	Antipsychotic	$4.4
Singulair	Oral asthma drug	$4.1
Crestor	Cholesterol-lowering drug	$3.8
Actos	Diabetes drug	$3.5
Epogen	Injectable anemia drug	$3.3

Instead of masking symptoms, we must start listening to them. Symptoms are the body's way of communicating with us. They are the red flags; they signal that things have gone awry and need to be restored as soon as possible! Remember, the body has a forgiving nature, but upset it too many times and frequent symptoms such as bloating, fatigue, joint pain and gas can develop into more serious health conditions and even disease processes.

Food fact: A recent study published in the *New England Journal of Medicine* found that even though liposuction removed up to 12 percent of body weight, it did not decrease the risk of heart disease or diabetes, as losing weight through diet and exercise does.

Quality of Life by Choice, Not Chance

"To wish to be well is a part of becoming well."

—Lucius Seneca

Of all the information in this book, this is probably the most important of all: The one factor that can make the greatest difference in your health and your looks is *you*! You are the gatekeeper to what you allow to filter in physically and mentally, and although you can obtain health coaches in the form of doctors, trainers and books, the key link is you. In order for you to get the most out of the 4-step program, I encourage you to really consider and be honest about your own current state of health. Think about where and how you would like to see improvements. Start this process by filling out the following brief medical history below:

1. When I get sick it is typically in my _____ system (refer to list below).

Examples of symptoms associated with various systems are:

Digestive system—gas, bloating, diarrhea, constipation, fatigue, yeast infections, excess weight, irritable bowel syndrome

Nervous system—numbness, tingling, headaches, anxiety attacks, depression, difficulty sleeping, lack of focus

Musculoskeletal system—stiffness, headaches, strains, sprains, lower back pain

Cardiovascular system—high or low blood pressure, high cholesterol, heart palpitations, heart disease

Immune system—frequent colds and flus, cold sores, sore throats, bronchitis, strep throat, sinusitis, yeast infections, allergies, asthma, chronic inflammation, fatigue

Endocrine system (includes pituitary gland, thyroid, parathyroid, thymus, adrenal glands, pancreas, ovaries and testes)—excess weight, excessive weight loss, difficulty sleeping, dry hair and skin, poor blood sugar control, fatigue, nervousness, poor libido

Reproductive system—painful menstruation, lack of menstruation, difficulty getting pregnant

Urinary system—urinary tract infections, frequent urination, involuntary urinary leakage

Lymphatic system—swollen glands, fatigue

Respiratory system—asthma, bronchitis, emphysema

2. I was sick _____ times last year.

3. I have been on medication ___100%___ times in the past year.

4. The part of my outer health and beauty I would like to change the most is (please list five goals in order of most importance to you, e.g., lose weight; achieve a radiant complexion; clear up acne or bags under my eyes; have shiny hair):
1. __lose weight__
2. __Kl news__
3. __bags under eyes.__
4. _____
5. _____

5. My energy level is __4__ out of 10 (10 being optimal energy; 1 being extremely low energy).

Now that you have identified your weakest system and the changes you would like to see happen, you have a reference point as you start or continue to climb the ladder towards internal health and external beauty. Review your recorded goals after 1 month, 3 months, 6 months and 1 year of following my program. I also recommend taking a "before" picture of yourself in order to notice the differences that are about to happen. Within a short time, you will be happily surprised to see how your primary health and beauty concerns have cleared up and your energy, vitality and pep in your step have markedly improved.

chapter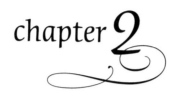

THE THREE BEAUTY ROBBERS

"The first wealth is health."
—RALPH WALDO EMERSON

From my experience in practice and from hours of pouring over nutritional research, I have been able to identify three main physiological processes that rob the body of inside health and outside beauty and vitality. Reversing the deteriorating effects of these processes and having them work in our favor allows health, wellness and a "natural pretty" to shine thru. The three beauty robbers are:

1. Faulty digestion
2. Chronic inflammation
3. Free radical damage

Figure 2.1: The Three Beauty Robbers

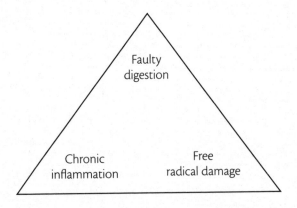

Beauty Robber #1 — Faulty Digestion

Although all systems are essential to the smooth functioning of the body, if there were to be a "master" system, it would be the digestive system. When dealing with any symptom or disease process, from eczema to heart disease, it is always critical to take a step back and investigate the overall health and integrity of an individual's digestive capacity. Start to consider the overall health of your digestive system by asking yourself the following questions. If you answer yes to one or more of the questions below, it is more than likely that your digestive system is in need of a tune-up.

- Do you suffer from heartburn? ✓
- Are you having irregular bowel movements (i.e., constipation or diarrhea)? *Loose*
- Do you have to strain to have a bowel movement?
- Are you having less than one bowel movement per day?
- Have you been on antibiotics in the last year?
- Have you suffered from yeast infections in the past?
- Do you frequently experience bloating follow-ing a meal?
- Do you feel tired after eating a meal?

When an individual's digestive capacity is compromised due to stress, faulty food choices, an overgrowth of yeast or parasites, a state of *dysbiosis* occurs. Dysbiosis is defined as the state where "friendly" bacteria or the microflora in the intestinal tract are upset and out of balance, leading to myriad health problems. In other words, without the proper "good bacteria" to keep your intestinal tract in check, the digestive system is unable to throw off toxins properly. Toxic build-up due to faulty digestion and elimination results in sickness in the area of your weakest link.

Your Pipes

The digestive system can be likened to an intricate pipeline system which starts at the mouth and ends at the anus. There are many physiological processes that take place in order to assimilate the minerals, vitamins and fiber from the sandwich you ate at lunch to fuel that will run your body. Although I am not going to bore you with a lengthy explanation on the biology or chemistry involved in digestion, I feel it's important to understand in brief how this system works.

The primary goal of the digestive system is to absorb and break down nutrients from foods into smaller molecules to be absorbed into the blood. For example, the macronutrients carbohydrates, fats and protein are broken down into:

- Proteins → amino acids
- Fats → fatty acids
- Carbohydrates → glucose

In addition, the digestive system is responsible for ridding the body of unwanted waste matter.

The digestive system, in turn, can be broken down into three primary actions:

1. **Secretion:** Enzymes' secretions are the catalysts that assist with the proper breakdown of food.
2. **Absorption:** Transport of water, ions and nutrients from the lumen and intestinal epithelium into the blood.
3. **Motility:** Contraction of smooth muscular wall (of the stomach) to crush, mix and expel the contents from the intestinal tract.

So, how does this pipeline work? Read on about the story of digestion to see where it all begins and ends. Refer to figure 2.2.

Nose: Surprisingly, the digestive system first begins in the nose! When the nose detects an appealing smell such as a fresh baked pie or a home-made meal, the brain is signaled to start releasing saliva in the mouth. This sparks the digestive system to start working and gets the body ready to break down the food it is about to receive.

Mouth: The mouth and teeth break down the food mechanically through the action of chewing and lubricating the food with saliva. An enzyme called *salivary amylase* is also secreted in the mouth which begins the breakdown of carbohydrates into smaller sugar units. The environment of the digestive system is measured by a scale called the potential of hydrogen (pH). This scale ranges from 0 to 14 with 1 being the most acidic and 14 the most alkaline. The pH of the mouth is alkaline. As you will discover in future chapters, in order to obtain internal health that translates into external vibrancy, it is crucial to keep your body fluids (with the exception of hydrochloric acid secreted from the stomach) slightly more alkaline.

Food Fact: Chewing your food properly is an essential part of digestion. With today's fast-paced lifestyles, a majority of people gulp down large amounts of food that have not been properly chewed. These undigested food particles are perceived as invaders and can trigger a negative reaction in the body such as inflammation, allergies, irritable bowel syndrome and constipation. The moral of the story: chew your food well!

Esophagus: After leaving the mouth, chewed-up food travels down a long tube called the esophagus in order to reach the stomach. At the junction of the esophagus and stomach, there is a ring-like valve closing the passage between the two organs. However, as the food approaches the closed ring, the surrounding muscles relax and allow the food to pass.

Stomach: The stomach secretes two critical components that continue the digestive process: the enzymes *pepsin* and *hydrochloric acid*. Pepsin is responsible for the breakdown of proteins such as those found in meat, chicken, dairy and eggs into smaller absorbable units called amino acids. Hydrochloric acid further assists with the breakdown of food and the absorption of minerals. In contrast to the mouth, the pH of the stomach is highly acidic; thus the stomach is lined with a mucus membrane for protection.

The stomach also performs a mechanical action by churning food into a liquid form called *chyme*. This step is necessary for the food's next stop in the small intestine.

Small intestine: The small intestine is a 20- to 22-foot-long tube and is lined with millions of *villi*, which move back and forth to absorb the broken down nutrients in your bloodstream. In fact, 99 percent of all absorption of nutrients occurs in the small intestine. The length of the small intestine is divided into three parts: the *duodenum*, the *jejunum* and the *ileum*. In the small intestine, the digestive juices once again switch to an alkaline state where protein, fats and carbohydrates are broken down. The pancreas provides a mixture of digestive enzymes to the small intestine which are critical for digestion of fats, carbohydrates and protein. The liver secretes bile salts into the small intestine, which are critical for digestion and absorption of fats. Bile acids dissolve fat into the watery contents of the small intestine, similar to the way detergents dissolve grease from a frying pan. Once the fat is dissolved, the enzyme mixture secreted by the pancreas digests the fat. Bile is stored in the gallbladder when not being utilized during mealtime.

Large intestine: The final stop on the food's journey down the intestinal tract ends in the large intestine and the rectum. The large intestine is five feet long and is divided into sections called the *cecum, ascending colon, transverse colon, descending colon, sigmoid colon* and *rectum*. The main function of the large intestine is healthy elimination. The large intestine contains "good bacteria" called microflora, which is crucial for proper digestion and elimination. In the large intestine, water is absorbed, bacterial fermentation takes place and feces are formed.

Figure 2.2: The Digestive System

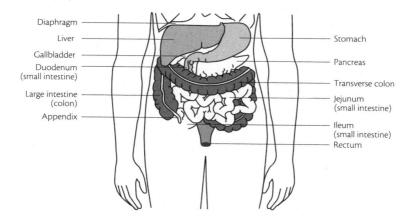

Figure 2.3: The Large Intestine

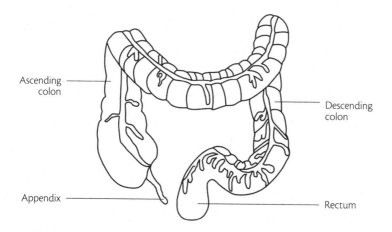

Food Facts: Time food spends in digestive system:
- Mouth: Seconds
- Esophagus: Seconds
- Stomach: Up to 3 ½ hours
- Small Intestine: Minutes
- Large Intestine: Hours

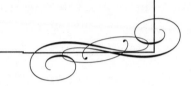

The Scoop on Poop

Let's be honest; this is not an easy topic to discuss. While many of us may be uncomfortable at the thought of talking about our bowel movements, they are a key component to health. One of the fastest ways to clear up skin and drop weight quickly is to clean up the digestive system. This is also the reason why you will find the first step in the program (chapter 3) beginning with a five-day detoxification plan. It is an "out with the bad, in with the good" approach to health that sets down the platform for healing and wellness.

WHAT IS NORMAL?

A person with a healthy functioning bowel should have a minimum of one well-formed bowel movement a day. For those with optimal functioning bowels, a normally formed bowel movement two to three times a day following each meal can be expected. Often, the intestinal tract becomes irritated due to the quality and quantity of food we are eating. Eating too late at night, consuming supersized meals and eating refined sugars, flours, trans fats and heavy proteins such as red meat clog up the pipes and suppress inner health and outer beauty from coming to fruition. Many people live with uncomfortable symptoms such as bloating, constipation and straining, thinking these symptoms are normal. They are not. A compromised digestive system will "spill over" into other areas of your health and can cause a multitude of symptoms such as headaches, fatigue, inflammation in your joints and skin problems.

Unfortunately, digestive diseases and disturbances are becoming more common. People suffering from Crohn's disease, colitis, irritable bowel syndrome, constipation, diarrhea, bloating and yeast infections frequently come into my office unsure of how to restore bowel health. Many are given the advice from their medical practitioner to simply increase their fiber in order to clear up the problem. Yet, increasing fiber alone will usually not do the trick. The key to digestive success is to address the underlying problem in the digestive tract, heal the irritated area and ensure proper absorption is taking place. Similar to a child's skinned knee that will be re-injured every time the child falls off his bike, every time a poor meal is eaten, it will cause irritation to the intestinal lining. This is also why simply improving the quality of nutrition often does not work if the problem has gone too far. Without even realizing it, many people's digestive systems take years of abuse. The symptoms they consider normal are the body's way of crying out, "I need some help over here!" The key is to heal and clean out the digestive system with essential fats, minerals and vitamins followed by an optimal diet and health plan. Turn to chapter 3 for how to optimize digestive health by beginning step 1—your five-day detoxification and cleanse.

WHAT'S SO BAD ABOUT YEAST?

Yeast, also called *candida albicans,* is a fungus that normally lives in our intestinal tract. A problem arises when the balance of yeast in our system increases, causing an overgrowth and crowding out of other friendly bacteria in our intestine. What was once harmless little yeast, overgrows and becomes aggressive and toxic. In fact, when yeast proliferates, its structure changes to one with root-like structures that penetrate the intestinal lining. The penetration of the intestinal lining allows unwanted invaders such as undigested food particles to enter and spill over into the bloodstream, creating toxic effects. It is as though tiny holes have been created in the barrier (the intestinal tract) that normally provides protection from foreign substances. The reaction to these invaders is the body's defense mechanism kicking in and often results in many health problems. This situation can also be referred to as "leaky gut syndrome."

While an overgrowth of yeast in an individual's system can be silent for long periods of time, as time goes on, it often becomes extremely troublesome, placing extreme stress on the person's overall health. Symptoms typically associated with an overgrowth of yeast include:

- Fatigue and general "fogginess"
- Depression, anxiety
- Pre-menstrual syndrome
- Cravings for sweets, alcohol and carbohydrates
- Headaches
- Yeast infections
- Difficulty losing weight
- Oral thrush (small white patches on the inside of the mouth)
- Constipation, bloating, abdominal pain
- Diarrhea

The two main circumstances that frequently create the environment for yeast to overgrow and develop into a state of *dysbiosis* (upset stomach flora) are:

1. The repeated or long-term use of antibiotics
2. A diet high in acid-forming foods (refined sugars and meats) and low in alkaline-forming foods (vegetables and most fruits)

Without clearing the yeast from an individual's system, achieving internal health is extremely difficult, if not impossible. In order to clear the yeast, the following steps must be taken:

1. Supplement with a high-quality probiotic daily such as acidophilus and bifidus.
2. Take a garlic supplement. Garlic has antifungal properties and can help kill the yeast.
3. Take a high-quality multi-vitamin and fish oil supplement to boost immunity.
4. Drink plenty of water to flush out your system.
5. Avoid sugars, alcohol and yeasty foods such as bread, rolls and pretzels.
6. Avoid fungus foods such as mushrooms.
7. Eliminate vinegar or foods that contain vinegar such as mustards, salad dressings, pickles and mayonnaise.
8. Eat plenty of fresh vegetables.
9. Consume yeast-free whole grains such as brown rice, millet, spelt, buckwheat and barley.
10. Consume a protein source such as fish, chicken or eggs at each and every meal.

Depending on the chronic nature of the yeast, it can often be extremely difficult to overcome. In addition to following the above recommendations, it is also best to seek the help of a naturopathic doctor or a healthcare practitioner familiar with treating yeast. To determine if you have an overgrowth of yeast in your system, a stool sample called the Comprehensive Digestive Stool Analysis (CDSA) can be taken and analyzed. This test is considered controversial by some medical doctors and is not standard. Even so, I feel it is a very important diagnostic tool to be considered as it can determine the possibility of parasites, candida and undigested proteins in your digestive system. I typically recommend this test only if individuals do not respond to dietary and supplement recommendations. For more information on doctors in your area who order CDSA, visit Great Smokies Laboratories at www.gsdl.com. Because becoming familiar with a yeast-free diet can feel overwhelming, I recommend *The Yeast Connection Cookbook* by William Crook for detailed dietary recommendations to clear up any confusion.

> **Food Fact:** Take your time when eating and relax! It takes a minimum of 20 minutes for the stretch receptors in the stomach to register a "full" or "satiated" signal in the brain.

Beauty Robber #2 — Chronic Inflammation

What do Type II diabetes, Alzheimer's disease, obesity, cancer, heart disease, stroke, Parkinson's and rheumatoid arthritis all have in common? Ground-breaking research indicates that they may all begin with an inflammatory process.

Inflammation is the body's first line of defense against harmful invaders such as unwanted bacteria, viruses and a multitude of other nasty critters. The inflammatory process has several soldiers in the form of white blood cells that act as protective agents when the body is attacked. Although this process is critical to maintaining the balance of health, researchers and scientist have now demonstrated that problems arise when the inflammatory process becomes chronic and no longer switches "off." In fact, hundreds of studies now pinpoint inflammation as the platform in which several disease processes begin such as heart disease, colon cancer and Alzheimer's disease.

The Western lifestyle, which includes fast foods, trans fats, smoking, lack of omega-3 essential fats and fresh produce in the diet and stress, promotes chronic inflammation. The stimulus that triggers the defense mechanism of inflammation to occur is either eaten, drunk or smoked by millions of people without realizing the underlying damage they are doing to their health. Simply because inflammation is not detected by a blood test, X-ray or other diagnostic measurement does not mean it is not occurring. On a microscopic level, inflammation can be silently and slowly wreaking havoc on your weakest link. From a beauty perspective, chronic inflammation can rob your looks by showing up as acne, eczema, bags under the eyes and difficulty losing weight. The good news is that given the proper environment and conditions—an alkaline environment with the proper foods and supplements—chronic inflammation can be prevented and even reversed. For more information, see chapter 3.

ON THE BATTLEFIELD

To understand inflammation, it is important to be aware of the cascade of events that takes place when the body is alerted there is a mini war to fight. This is referred to as *innate immunity*—the body's unique and mysterious ability to heal a wound or fight off an invader when trouble arises. What is perceived as "trouble" to the body can appear in the form of numerous agents such as bacteria, viruses, "bad fats," too much white sugar, stress or environmental toxins such as herbicides and pesticides. In short, the key role of in-flammation is to attack and repair. To understand how this process works, let's take the example of a young boy falling off his bike and scraping his knee. In response to potential bacteria entering the cut in his knee, a type of cell called mast cells are signaled to release histamine and cytokines to create tiny leaks in blood vessel walls. The leaks allow other immune cells to rush to the battlefield. At the same time, a large cell called the macrophage starts an attack on bacteria and other unwanted chemicals by secreting harmful toxins to "kill off" the bad guys. Finally, another type of specialized white blood cell called the neutrophil engulfs and destroys the bacteria while other lymphocytes (white blood cells) work actively to boost immune system function. If necessary, the body will then form a clot to heal the wound. Presto—wound healed, scab formed and the young boy's knee will be good as new in five to 10 days. The process looks like this:

Figure 2.4: The Inflammatory Process

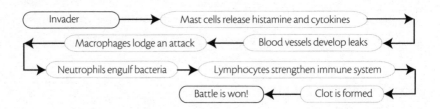

So, why is it thought that inflammation is the underlying cause of serious disease processes such as heart disease, stroke and cancer? Remember, inflammation is not the problem; in fact, it is an incredibly adaptive response we need to survive. The problem is when the switch does not get turned off and chronic inflammation develops and ensues.

NOT JUST AN "ITIS"

In school, we were always taught that anything that ended in "itis" indicated an inflammatory response such as bronchitis (inflammation of the bronchioles), colitis (inflammation of the colon) and sinusitis (inflammation of the sinus tracts). When dealing with the conventional medical model, an "itis" is typically treated with an anti-inflammatory and/or pain medication. Unfortunately, many of these medications have mild to severe side effects. The term "side effect" in reference to a drug has always been curious to me. From my perspective, all effects of a drug, whether termed side effect or not, should be considered on an equal scale. After all effects are made known to consumers/patients, they then make the decision to take or not to take the medication.

> In 2004, a very commonly prescribed anti-inflammatory drug, Vioxx (by Merck and Co.)—known as a COX-2 inhibitor, used to treat arthritis and acute pain—was recalled due to its risk of causing heart complications. Vioxx was one of Merck's most lucrative drugs, with $2.5 billion in sales in 2003.

In addition to the side effects of anti-inflammatory drugs, there are other concerns. If the inflammatory process is being suppressed by an intervention such as a medication, the once protective response of the body is being forced off. Of course, if there is chronic inflammation that is creating a dangerous situation, there are times when this may be necessary. However, once the drug is removed, the body often experiences a "rebound effect." In other words, the body says, "Aha, the drug is not suppressing me anymore, so I can create a situation that promotes even more inflammation!" Oftentimes, if the drugs are not prescribed long term and the patient stops using them, symptoms will worsen. For example, colitis patients may experience a "flare-up" in their condition or individuals suffering from "frozen shoulder" will feel more stiffness and pain once they stop their anti-inflammatory medication. Doesn't it make far more sense to deal with the cause of the underlying inflammatory response, rather than merely silencing it?

By following the 4-step program outlined in chapters 3–6, the stimulus (trans fats, smoking, stress, poor diet) that causes chronic inflammation will be removed and will be replaced with natural anti- inflammatory foods and supplements. What is an anti-inflammatory food? It is a food source that not only prevents chronic inflammation from occurring, but can also reverse the process once it has started. As you will see in the following pages and in the delicious recipes at the end of the book, anti-inflammatory foods can be tasty and incredibly nutritious at the same time. In addition to preventing the diseases dominating in North America today such as cancer, heart disease, stroke and arthritis, eating anti-inflammatory foods will also prevent wrinkles, prevent weight gain, make hair shiny and soft and give you a glowing and radiant complexion.

Beauty Robber #3 — Free Radical Damage

In order to understand free radical damage, a very brief lesson in chemistry is required. All cells in the body are composed of several different types of molecules. Molecules are composed of one or more smaller units called atoms. Atoms contain several parts including a nucleus, neutrons, protons and electrons. Electrons are negatively charged and protons are positively charged. Electrons orbit around the atom in one or more rings. The atom is stable when the electron ring is full. For example, when the innermost electron ring has two electrons, it is full and moves to the second ring. When the second electron ring has eight electrons, it is full and moves on to another ring and so on (see figure 2.5). Free radical damage occurs when one of the rings of the atom does not have a full set of electrons and is therefore unstable. In order to find stability, the atom will literally rip another electron from a neighboring cell to take it as its own. The "ripping" or "stealing" of a neighboring electron from the cell's membrane creates damage and destruction to the cell called free radical damage. Unfortunately, this domino effect creates a dangerous chain reaction creating more and more damaged cells.

Figure 2.5: Free Radical Damage

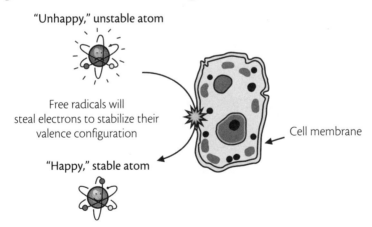

"Unhappy," unstable atom

Free radicals will steal electrons to stabilize their valence configuration

Cell membrane

"Happy," stable atom

Free radical damage can be caused by many factors including invading bacteria, viruses or by-products of metabolism. However, similar to the other two beauty robbers, faulty digestion and chronic inflammation, the Western lifestyle is a major contributor to chronic free radical damage and cellular destruction. Environmental factors such as lack of fruits and vegetables in the diet, smoking, stress, herbicides and pesticides all create "rips" in cellular membranes.

Similar to inflammation, a certain amount of free radical damage is normal and expected. From the thoughts we think, to the food we eat and water we drink, our cells are constantly bombarded with "mini hits" from the environment. However, when we tip the scales too much in the wrong direction by taking in too much of the "bad stuff" and too little of the "good stuff," free radical damage occurs, stealing our health and robbing our beauty.

Figure 2.6: Tipping the Scale on Free Radical Damage

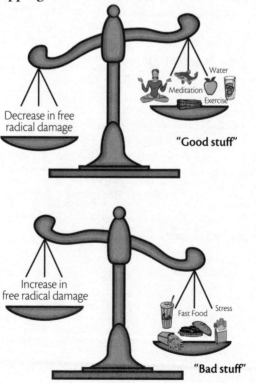

ANTIOXIDANTS—THE NEUTRALIZERS

As scientists and doctors now know, cellular damage, such as that created by free radical damage, is one of the underlying causes of illnesses and disease. However, given the proper antioxidants, cells can be repaired and disease processes can be prevented and reversed. Specifically, antioxidants in the diet such as vitamins A, C and E, superoxide dismutase, flavonoids, beta carotene, glutathione, selenium and zinc can all neutralize free radical damage.

Now that you have an understanding of the three beauty robbers—1) Faulty digestion, 2) Inflammation and 3) Free radical damage—you have an understanding of the physiological processes that rob your health and steal your beauty. The rest of the book will provide you with the steps on how to halt and reverse these processes to look and feel your best. In other words, by optimizing digestion, preventing and minimizing inflammation and counteracting and balancing free radical damage, you will be on the path to optimal health, weight loss and beauty.

Are you ready to start the program? Let's begin.

chapter 3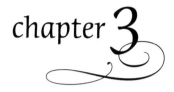

STEP 1— YOUR FIVE-DAY CLEANSE

"A man too busy to take care of his health is like a mechanic too busy to take care of his tools."

—SPANISH PROVERB

Getting into the Health Groove

Step 1 consists of a five-day detoxifying and cleansing period that is crucial for the body. When starting any health program, it is always best to begin with a gentle cleanse to get rid of unwanted "internal garbage." By doing this, you are allowing your body to set the stage for healing to take place and natural beauty to emerge. Where does internal garbage come from? There are several practices that contribute to the beauty robbers mentioned in the previous chapters. The top 10 things that rob health and fill up your body with unwanted waste are:

1. Eating refined white flour and sugary foods
2. Dehydration (excess coffee and alcohol intake, lack of fresh, clean water)
3. Consumption of trans fats
4. Lack of omega-3 essential fats in the diet
5. Lack of anti-inflammatory foods in the diet
6. Smoking
7. Stress
8. Lack of exercise
9. Repetitive use of antibiotics
10. Poor sleeping patterns

Some people may have one of the above health robbers in their lives, while others have many. By following the cleanse outlined in this chapter, you will give your body the opportunity for wellness and vitality to emerge.

You Gotta Wanna!

It is estimated that over 50 percent of all the leading killers in women, including heart disease, lung cancer, stroke, breast cancer, obesity and depression are related to behavior. In other words, change your behavior and your chance of survival will increase dramatically. I realize as adults, we are set in our ways and change can often feel challenging or difficult. Excuses such as, "I don't have enough time," "I don't have enough money," or "I am a picky eater," seem to take precedence over us doing something good for our health. Alternatively, there are many who have tried the latest health programs and diet fads only to fail and become even more frustrated. Who wouldn't give up with repeated attempts that end up as an exercise in futility? I recognize all of these factors and witness them in practice daily. I also realize that change has to be realistic, motivating, easy to implement into a busy life and offer dramatic health and beauty results. This is the reason I begin the Natural Makeover Diet with the five-day cleanse. By cleansing you set the stage for dramatic results and healing to occur. After the five days, you will find the nutritional, supplement and lifestyle recommendations realistic, long lasting and energizing. However, as the comedian Steve Martin has been quoted saying, "You gotta wanna." Similar to not being able to force a smoker to quit, the time has to be right for you. The good news is, the fact that you are reading this passage at this very moment likely means you are motivated for change and ready to start taking charge of your inner health and outer beauty. Change begins with intention and initiative, so the desire must come from within.

I highly recommend strictly sticking to the five-day cleanse in order to reap the best results. After that, I recommend the 80–20 rule of health. In other words, eat, sleep and move in a healthy manner 80 percent of the time and allow yourself the grace of falling off the health wagon 20 percent of the time (on weekends and holidays and at parties). If you fall off the health wagon from time to time (and I actually encourage it!), do not panic or be hard on yourself. By following the guidelines in this book, you will be able to indulge some of the time, all the while maintaining your health goals. The only exception to this rule is if you are suffering from a chronic illness, are in chronic pain or have food intolerances. In those situations, strict dietary adherence is required at all times.

Although changing your behavior is critical, my objective in writing this book is not focused simply on survival or prevention of disease. By following the program, you will propel your current level of health and will experience the look and feel of what I refer to as "getting into your own health groove." The health groove is a zone that feels different for everyone. Once in the health groove, there will be a certain energy about you, a certain glow that is almost indescribable, making you look and feel your best. Depending on your "weakest link," you will see improvements in different areas. You may notice instant results in your skin or will quickly drop 5 to 10 pounds. Or you may notice a decrease in bloating after meals. Most of you will also feel a natural high that can only be achieved by eating specific foods. Instead of dragging your feet out of bed in the morning with stiff joints and tired eyes and skin, you will have a vigor that translates into all areas of your life, including your mood, body weight, outside appearance and internal health.

You may feel skeptical that a five-day cleanse period is long enough to effect change, but I assure you, it is. Remember, the body has an amazing forgiving nature and when given the proper nourishment, you will notice a response in a very short time.

To Fast or Not to Fast?

I am often asked if it is best to fast during a cleanse for a certain time period (one, three or five days). My response to this question for the most part is "no." There are several reasons why fasting is not a good idea. First, due to the overprocessing of our grains and sugar, lack of fiber and a sedentary lifestyle, millions of North Americans are walking around with a syndrome called *metabolic syndrome*. Although it is now estimated that one out of every five Americans has this syndrome, because it often goes undiagnosed, the numbers are likely significantly higher. Metabolic syndrome is a collection of health risks that increase your chance of developing heart disease, stroke and diabetes. The condition is also known by other names including *syndrome X, insulin resistance syndrome* and *dysmetabolic syndrome*. In short, those with metabolic syndrome do not have proper blood sugar or insulin control. Fasting would likely send these individuals into a state of hypoglycemia (low blood sugar), making them feel extremely shaky, fatigued and dizzy with the possibility of fainting. How do you know if you may suffer from metabolic syndrome? Ask yourself the following questions:

- Do you feel shaky from meal to meal?
- Do you experience intense food or sugar cravings?
- Do you experience high and low energy surges throughout the day?
- Do you have a history of heart disease or Type II diabetes in your family?
- Are you overweight?
- Do you have difficulty losing weight?

If you have answered yes to one or more of these questions, it is advisable to visit your doctor to have your blood sugars checked. For more details on the interaction between food, insulin and fat, refer to chapter 4.

The second reason why I do not recommend fasting is due to an adaptive response called "*the starvation adaptation mode.*" Starvation adaptation mode occurs when the body's caloric intake is severely restricted or, in the case of a fast, completely absent. When this occurs, the brain gets the message that it is undergoing a time of famine. As a safety measure and as a prehistoric response that dates back to the time when famines were a reality, the body holds on to fat for protection. In other words, when calories are limited or when there are no calories consumed at all, the body attempts to hold on to its weight. Even worse for weight loss seekers, once they begin consuming more calories, the body thinks, "Aha! Here is some food. I better store it as fat in case of a future emergency." That's fairly counterproductive when it comes to weight loss, isn't it? This is one of the main reasons why diets that severely restrict calories (under 800 calories per day) will always result in failure.

The key to a successful program is to begin with a gentle cleanse, not a fast. By doing so, you will support the detoxification process, all the while getting yourself to the next rung on the ladder of health. Do not worry about counting calories or grams of carbohydrates, proteins or fat while on your five-day cleanse. Simply follow the guidelines outlined below.

The Herxheimer Reaction

When undergoing any type of detoxification process or cleanse, an unpleasant side effect called the Herxheimer reaction is unlikely but can occur. According to Dorland's medical dictionary, "The reaction has been attributed to liberation of endotoxin-like substances or of antigens from the killed or dying microorganisms." Simply put, the body is detoxifying at such a rapid rate that toxins are being "killed off" faster than the body can eliminate them. Often individuals describe this reaction as the feeling of getting worse before getting better or as a "fluish feeling." Symptoms of the Herxheimer reaction can include fatigue, a white coating on the tongue, head-aches, moodiness and either constipation or diarrhea. Although this reaction may not occur during your five-day cleanse, if it does, don't give up; you are merely cleaning up your "internal garbage." There are many steps that can be taken to minimize the effects.

- Drink water with fresh-squeezed lemon.
- Eat raw fruits and vegetables for fiber.
- Add flaxseeds to a morning shake to ensure your bowels are moving.
- Exercise and stretch.
- If weather permits, get your dose of sunshine.

As with all diets and cleanses, the five-day cleanse is not recom-mended if you are pregnant or breastfeeding.

Dealing with Cravings

> "The definition of craving: an intense desire for some par-ticular thing."
>
> —*Webster's* dictionary

In addition to the Herxheimer reaction, many people report that the reason they fall off the health wagon and resort to their old ways is due to intense cravings for sweets or carbohydrates such as chocolate, breads or bagels. I often hear people say, "I need to eat something sweet after each meal." Similar to a craving for a drink or a cigarette, food cravings are powerful chemical messages from the brain that can be extremely intense and difficult to fight off. More often than not, trying to resist the urge to satisfy a craving usually results in failure. Like an addiction, the message sent from the brain for a sweet or a starchy carbohydrate occurs at a biochemical level and is very real. Instead of trying to resist the urge, the key to getting rid of your cravings is to clean up your act nutritionally. Pay attention to your cravings. They are one of the best indicators that you are consuming too many refined and processed foods and not taking in sufficient amounts of vitamins, minerals, essential fats and water. How do you know if you have cravings or suffer from what I refer to as "sweet tooth syndrome"? Next time you want a sweet or starchy food, examine the feeling you are experiencing before you indulge. Do you feel "I would like to eat that chocolate chip cookie," or is your feeling more intense such as "I cannot focus on anything else until I eat that chocolate chip cookie!"?

Most cravings are due to fluctuating blood sugar levels. As will be explained in more detail in chapter 4, when a diet consists of refined foods such as muffins, processed breads and pastas, coffee, white sugar and pop, your blood sugar undergoes a constant roller-coaster ride. When you have low blood sugar (hypoglycemia), which can occur anywhere from 20 minutes to three hours after your last meal or snack, you will feel foggy, tired, moody and perhaps even shaky. In order to counteract these uncomfortable symptoms, the brain will signal a craving to eat something sweet or starchy to bring up blood sugar levels. Although this will take care of the problem temporarily, it results in an up-and-down vicious cycle of cravings and weight gain.

When you eat the right type of protein, fats and fiber in proper balance and take in the proper minerals, vitamins and supplements, you will no longer experience intense cravings. You will be able to eat the occasional sweet treat without falling back into your unhealthy eating patterns that consist of sugar, refined carbohydrates, coffee and pop. Remember, it is a good idea to indulge once in a while—I recommend it! Constant deprivation is a one-way ticket to failure. However, any food item that is unhealthy can always be made in a healthier form. All you have to do is learn the nutritional tricks of the trade and apply them to your lifestyle. Refer to the recipe section at the back of this book for balanced, nutritious and delicious meals and snacks.

During the five-day cleanse, your cravings may appear to be heightened and more intense. This is normal and will subside by the second week of the program. In order to curb your response of grabbing a sugary or grainy treat when you are in the throws of a craving, I recommend the following steps to get you over the hump:

1. Drink plenty of water with fresh-squeezed lemon.
2. Drink sweet berry herbal teas.
3. Take chewable vitamin C—500–1000 mg at a time.
4. Experiment with natural sweeteners such as stevia that do not alter blood sugar levels.
5. Eat one or two Dr. Joey's Skinnychews, which are naturally sweetened, dark-chocolate chews with 4 grams of prebiotic inulin fiber per serving. With fewer than 20 calories per chew, they are the perfect option for 3 p.m. cravings or nighttime eating. For more information, please visit www.drjoey.com.
6. If cravings are severe, consider supplementing with a chromium supplement, available at all health food stores.

Acid versus Alkaline

Balanced body chemistry is of the utmost importance for the maintenance of health and the prevention of disease. The ideal body chemistry is slightly more alkaline. Unfortunately, the majority of people have overly acidic body chemistry due to poor food choices such as red meats, refined sugars and flours and excessive dairy and alcohol consumption. In addition, research shows that North Americans are consuming too few alkaline-forming foods in the form of vegetables, fruits and whole grains. When the body is overly acidic, it creates an opportune environment for disease, infection and inflammation to occur. In addition, in an attempt to return to a more alkaline state, the body will seek out a buffer to counteract the acidity. Calcium, the most abundant alkaline (a.k.a. basic) mineral in the body is leached from the bones in an attempt to maintain normal body chemistry. This is one of the theories as to why North Americans, one of the largest dairy consumers in the world, also suffer from the greatest amount of osteoporosis (bone loss). Overindulgence in acid-forming foods such as dairy, refined flours and meat, caffeine and soda pop will eventually create a calcium deficit.

All foods are burned in the body, leaving behind an ash residue that is either acidic or alkaline, depending on the mineral composition of the food. To prevent disease and to look and feel your best, the body should be slightly more alkaline than acidic. In other words, 70 to 80 percent of the food you eat should be derived from alkaline-forming foods such as leafy greens, most fruits, soy products and seeds; only 20 to 30 percent should be derived from acid-forming foods such as grains, red meat and dairy products. By eating within this ratio, the body is protected from a state of acidosis. In reality, the North American diet has this ratio backwards, consuming approximately 20 percent of the diet from alkaline foods and the remainder from acid-forming foods.

The scale used to measure the acid/alkaline balance in the body is called the pH scale (potential of hydrogen). The normal pH level of saliva ranges from 6.8 to 7. A higher level shifts you to a more alkaline state and a lower level shifts you to a more acidic state. In order to test your own pH, you can simply purchase pH paper from your local health food store. For best results, test your pH two hours before or after a meal. Use a 1-inch-long piece of pH paper. If testing with urine, put the pH paper in contact with the urine midstream or into a cup containing a urine sample. If using saliva, do not let the strip touch your tongue or mouth. Rather, collect a sample of saliva in a spoon or cup and dip the pH paper in. Once the paper makes contact with the urine or saliva, immediately compare the color of the pH paper with the color-coded chart that comes along with the pH kit. Write down your results and test once or twice per week for a 30-day period to watch a shift in color occur as you become more alkaline. Yellowish green is more on the acidic side while bluish green is closer to an alkaline state. Please refer to the appendix for a list of alkaline- and acid-forming foods.

The 4-step program outlined in *The Natural Makeover Diet* is designed to gradually and naturally shift you towards a more alkaline state. If you received an acidic reading, test again within two to four weeks to see your results and improvement.

Beginning the Five-Day Cleanse

> *"When health is absent*
> *Wisdom cannot reveal itself,*
> *Art cannot be exerted,*
> *Wealth is useless and Reason is powerless."*
> —Herophilies, 300 B.C.

Now that you have an understanding of why cleansing is important and the symptoms that you may or may not experience, you are ready to begin. Remember, you may panic at first and think, "There is no way I can give up all of my favorite foods!" Fear not, it is only for a five-day period and there are plenty of delicious and healthy options to choose from (see the five-day meal plan at the end of the chapter). The following chapters will provide you with details about how to eat healthier grains, sweets and other treats once your cleanse is complete without robbing your health or beauty. Remember, the five-day cleanse is done on its own, while steps two, three and four are done at the same time and can be maintained for life. I highly recommend referring to the food diary outlined in the appendix and recording all of your food for five days. Filling out the food journal will definitely help you to monitor your progress, your symptoms and your energy level.

The eight elements to the five-day cleanse are:

1. Eliminate all grains (including gluten-free grains).
2. Eliminate all dairy products (with the exception of 1 ounce of goat cheese per day).
3. Eliminate all red meat.
4. Eliminate all white sugar.
5. Take a minimum of three capsules of "friendly bacteria" (probiotic capsules or powder) daily with food.
6. Increase consumption of phytonutrient-rich foods, such as broccoli, kale, spinach, blueberries and raspberries.
7. Drink eight glasses of water or herbal tea daily (no juice, pop, coffee or alcohol).
8. Consume 1 tbsp. of ground flaxseeds daily and 2 to 3 grams of distilled fish oil.

Read on to find out the details of each step. In addition, refer to the back of the chapter for a sample meal plan for your five-day cleanse.

Element #1—Eliminate All Grains (including gluten-free grains)

In addition to consuming too many grains, North Americans also consume the wrong type of grain. The type and amount of grain you eat has a huge impact on health, body weight and appearance. Unfortunately, the stripping of whole grains down to white, refined floury products for breads, pasta, crackers, muffins and other grainy products is a common and economical practice followed by most food processors. Even bread that is marketed as "whole wheat" can be derived from refined flour. Some manufacturers simply add a bit of blackstrap molasses to the bread to make it appear brown. Tricky isn't it? Along with removing precious fiber, nutrients and fat, refined floury products are a one-way ticket to myriad health problems, including weight gain, fatigue, moodiness, hypoglycemia, digestive disorders, bloating and skin problems. In order to know if the next loaf of bread you purchase is a good type to buy, there are a couple of tests it should pass. First, when reading the label, check for the words "made from 100% whole wheat or whole grain." If you see the words *refined*, *white* or *processed* on the label, you know that the flour has been refined. The second test is to pick up the loaf of bread and squeeze it. Can you accordion the bread down to half of its size because it is so fluffy and light? If so, you are dealing with a refined product. Whole grain bread actually feels slightly heavier and grainier and cannot be squeezed down to half its size. To learn more, refer to page 190 to read about my bread test.

During the five-day cleanse, all grainy products should be removed in order to give your digestive system a break. Think of this process as a vacation for digestion and a chance to remove any of the abuse the body has endured in the past days, months or years. Grain products to be removed are:

- All breads, bagels, rolls, buns, wraps, croutons
- Pasta, pizza
- Crackers, muffins, cookies, cakes, granola bars, cereal, cereal bars
- Pretzels
- Oatmeal
- Rice

I find as we age, our ability to digest wheat and gluten products in large quantities tends to decrease. Part of this has to do with the control of our blood sugars and the other part has to do with digestion and inflammation. As you will see in the pages of this book, I am not a "no grain" nutritionist. However, I do recommend minimal grain intake (one to two servings per day before 3 p.m.) as we age to avoid middle-age spread, fatigue and cravings. With that said, the fiber (soluble and insoluble) in whole grains is invaluable, and that is why there is indeed a time and a place for them. In addition to the above grains, you should not consume white potatoes.

Table 3.1

Grain Listings	Is It Good for Your Health?
100% whole wheat or whole grain	Yes! This is a good option and refers to the fact that the entire grain (with all the nutrition) has been left intact. The three parts of a grain are: 1) the bran, 2) the germ and 3) the endosperm.

Wheat or wheat flour, semolina, durum wheat, organic flour, multigrain	Maybe. While these words offer accurate descriptions, they do not necessarily imply that the grain is intact.
Enriched	No! This word implies that the grain has been processed.

Element # 2 — Eliminate All Dairy Products

Dairy products derived from cow's milk are significantly more protein-dense in comparison to human milk. In fact, cow's milk derives 15 percent of its calories from protein, whereas in human milk, protein accounts for only 5 percent. The large percentage of proteins in cow's milk, specifically a protein called casein, can contribute to inflammation and digestive disturbances. Problems arise when the proteins in cow's milk are interpreted as invaders and attacked by the body. Your weakest link will determine where the attack will occur. This is also why cow's milk is considered one of the most allergenic foods consumed. Most people are led to believe they are lactose intolerant when, in fact, it is the proteins they are reacting to. How do you know if it is the proteins or the lactose (milk sugar) causing your symptoms? Switch to lactose-free milk and see if your symptoms subside. If not, it is likely the proteins in dairy products that are creating your uncomfortable symptoms. If this is the case, switching to a dairy-free diet is best (see table 3.2 for dairy-free calcium sources).

Not all people react to dairy, but if you do, symptoms may include asthma, allergies, acne, eczema, irritable bowel disorder, constipation, bloating, ear infections, sinusitis, chest infections, chronic runny nose, weight gain, fatigue, diarrhea and dark circles under the eyes.

In chapter 4, I will outline healthier dairy products that can be consumed in moderation.

To avoid any inflammation, all dairy products are to be removed from the diet during the five-day cleanse period, with the exception of goat cheese. Goat cheese is a highly digestible dairy option that can help to flavor meals. One ounce per day is permitted. (One ounce = the size of an average lipstick.)

Dairy products to be eliminated are:

- All cheeses (hard cheese, cream cheese)
- Milk
- Ice cream, frozen yogurt
- Yogurt
- Dips made with dairy
- Puddings
- Any other product that may contain casein (check label)

Table 3.2: Milligrams of Calcium in Non-Dairy Food Sources

Food Source	Milligrams of Calcium
1 cup of sesame seeds	2200 mg
Fortified ready-to-eat cereals (1 ounce)	236–1043 mg
1 cup of almonds	600 mg
1 cup of soybeans	460 mg
8-ounce glass of calcium-fortified orange juice	300 mg
1 cup of soy milk beverage original enriched	300 mg
1 cup of sunflower seeds	260 mg
3 ounces of salmon	203 mg

½ cup of collards	179 mg
1 cup of broccoli	178 mg
2-ounce piece of cornbread	133 mg
½ cup of frozen spinach	130 mg
1 package of instant oatmeal	100 mg

Element #3 — Eliminate All Red Meat

The inflammatory fats found in red meat have been linked to several disease processes including colon cancer and heart disease (refer to table 3.3 for examples of the amount of fat found in red meat products). In addition, red meat is acidic, steering the body away from the healthy alkaline state necessary for achieving internal health. Red meat is also extremely taxing on digestion and can take hours to digest. Keep in mind that in order to achieve the external state of beauty we are striving for, it is necessary to make our digestive system a fine working piece of equipment.

Red meats to be removed from the diet during the five-day cleanse include:

- Steak
- Bacon
- Cold cuts
- Ham
- Hamburgers
- Hot dogs
- Ribs
- Pork
- Veal

Although some people consider pork or veal a white, leaner meat, it is actually quite fatty and should be eliminated.

The protein sources recommended during the five-day cleanse are:

- Egg whites and/or whole eggs
- Protein powder—brown rice, pea or hemp
- 4–6 ounces of cold-water fish such as wild salmon, light tuna, mackerel
- 4–6 ounces of chicken or turkey
- 4–6 ounces of tofu per day or ½ cup of beans per day

Bean options include lentils, black beans, chickpeas, kidney beans or edamame. Please soak your beans overnight to aid with digestibility or purchase low-sodium beans. Keep in mind—half a cup only!

Table 3.3: Fat Grams in Food Items

Food Item	Total Fat	Total Saturated Fat
4 ounces of sirloin steak	15 grams	6 grams
4 ounces of pork spareribs	20 grams	8 grams
4 ounces of chicken breast	10 grams	3 grams
4 ounces of turkey breast	8 grams	2 grams
4 ounces of salmon fillet	4 grams	0 grams
1 veggie burger patty	4 grams	1 gram

Element #4 — Eliminate All White Sugar

White sugar is often the thorn in many chronic dieters' side. Many have tried to give up white sugary treats, only to be thrown into the roller-coaster ride of cravings, late-night munching and mood swings. If this sounds familiar, just follow the steps outlined in this chapter and your vicious cycle of sweet tooth syndrome will finally be broken!

White sugar is problematic on a number of levels. It causes blood sugar to bounce around, oversecretes insulin, causes weight gain, allows the overgrowth of yeast in the digestive system, increases acidity, creates dental cavities and causes fluctuations in our energy and mood. One of the most serious effects is that white sugar significantly suppresses immune system function. In other words, if we are fighting a "bug" or are in a time of stress and consume white sugar such as a can of pop, we leave our system wide open to sickness.

In order to measure the effect white sugar has on the body, a scale used to measure our white blood cell count (cells that fight infection) called the leukocytic index is used. The average leukocytic index is approximately 13.9. However, within 15 minutes of eating approximately 100 grams of refined sugar (i.e., a large 32-ounce Coke contains 90 grams of sugar), the leukocytic index drops to 1.9. In other words, we lose over 90 percent of our immune function following consumption of white sugary treats!

Most refined and processed goodies such as pop, cookies, crackers, cereal, ketchup, granola bars, yogurt and chocolate milk contain white sugar. In order to determine if a product contains white sugar, check the label. Labels list ingredients in descending order by weight. If a product's first ingredient is sugar, the percentage of sugar in that product is greater than any other, leaving little room for optimal nutrition. The following words indicate the presence of sugar in a food: *glucose, sucrose, fructose, high fructose corn syrup, white sugar, brown sugar, granulated sugar, powdered sugar, icing sugar* and *dextrose*.

For the five-day cleanse, it is best to eliminate sugar completely. Here's what is allowed during the five days:

- A maximum of two servings of fruit per day (serving size = 1 small fruit or ½ cup of sliced fruit). Make one of those selections berries such as blueberries, strawberries, raspberries or cranberries in a morning shake.

- Watered-down juice to help you get rid of cravings (¾ water, ¼ juice).
- 1 teaspoon of honey or maple syrup daily to sweeten herbal tea or a shake.
- 1–2 Dr. Joey's Skinnychews per day. If you put them in the freezer, they will last in your mouth longer. Visit www.drjoey.com.

The following chapters will review healthier sweet options and the safety of sugar substitutions.

Food Fact: The average American consumes approximately 20 teaspoons of sugar per day. A can of 12-ounce pop contains approximately 10 teaspoons (or 40 grams!) of sugar.

Element #5 — Take a Minimum of Three Capsules of "Friendly Bacteria" Daily

When most people think of bacteria, a negative image is conjured in their minds. Society's obsession with killing off bacteria is evidenced by our chronic use of antibiotics and antibacterial soaps. Yet, not all bacteria are bad. In fact, certain bacteria are considered "friendly" and are an integral part of health. These types of bacteria, called *probiotics*, normally inhabit our digestive system and are critical to the proper balance of our digestive *microflora* (the healthy bacteria that lives in our large intestine).

When processed foods are eaten in excess, or antibiotics are taken repetitively or during times of stress, our bodies become more acidic and digestive microflora suffers. When this happens, the "bad" bacteria in our gut can overpower our "friendly bacteria" allowing the overgrowth of yeast, parasites and many other nasty bugs. Because we are only as healthy as our digestive systems, an overgrowth of bad bugs manifests symptoms in other areas of our bodies. These include skin problems, fatigue, headaches and systemic yeast.

In order to clean sweep digestion, it is important to supplement with the friendly bacteria called *probiotics*. Acidophilus is one type of the friendly bacteria that can help to keep the harmful bacteria in check. The benefits of probiotics include:

- Improving digestive function
- Acting as a natural digestive aid that can be used for indigestion and upset stomach
- Killing off harmful bacteria and yeast
- Producing the enzyme lactase, which aids the digestion of milk products for those who are lactose intolerant
- Producing B vitamins and vitamin K in the body
- Assisting with bad breath
- Lowering cholesterol
- Promoting immune system functioning
- Helping to clear up skin problems such as acne

Probiotics are often sold in mixed-strain preparations that combine various species. Visit your local health food store to purchase an active culture that contains no fewer than 5–10 billion organisms per pill. Store probiotics in the refrigerator at all times.

During the five-day cleanse, I recommend taking a minimum of three capsules of probiotics per day with food. Following the cleanse, 1–2 capsules of probiotics per day for maintenance and optimal digestion is recommended.

Element #6 — Increase Consumption of Phytonutrient-Rich Foods

In the last decade of nutritional research, plant compounds called *phytonutrients* have been receiving more attention due to their powerful effect on health. Phytonutrients are found mostly in fruits, vegetables and to a lesser degree in soy and whole grains. They are responsible for giving many fruits and vegetables their color, hue, scent and flavor. Unlike a lack of minerals or vitamins, a lack of phytonutrients does not appear to create a deficiency syndrome, such as rickets (lack of vitamin D) or scurvy (lack of vitamin C). Yet, these powerful compounds offer extremely potent protection against a multitude of diseases. Research is now demonstrating that phytonutrients act as potent antioxidants that can neutralize free radical damage. In other words, they work to repair cells that have been damaged. Thus, by repairing cellular damage, inflammation is reduced, which causes skin to look its best. It is not unusual for my clients to soon notice a reduction in redness, dark circles and fine lines once a large amount of phytonutrients is introduced.

Food Fact: According to the American Dietetic Association, phytonutrients are associated with the prevention and/or treatment of four of the leading causes of death in the United States: cancer, diabetes, cardiovascular disease and hypertension.

In order to reach a state of inner health that translates into outer beauty, it is important to minimize the effects of free radical damage.

Consuming an abundant amount of phytonutrient-rich food daily is by far the most effective method to limit the damage. This step is critical while you are flushing out your system.

So, the question is, how much and what type of phytonutrient foods should you eat?

In terms of fruits, berries are the top choice as they are packed full of phytonutrients called *bioflavonoids* and are lower in sugar. You should eat one selection of berries (raspberries, blueberries, straw-berries or cranberries) daily, either on their own or in a shake (see page 85 for a delicious shake recipe). Remember: on the cleanse, 2 to 3 servings of fruit are allowed per day.

In terms of vegetables, the more the merrier. It is recommended that you consume a minimum of five servings of vegetables each day. A serving of vegetables is equal to:

- 1 cup of leafy vegetables such as spinach or let-tuce
- ½ cup of other cooked vegetables such as carrots or greens beans
- ¾ cup of vegetable juice

Some vegetables rich in phytonutrients are:

Asparagus	Tomatoes	Kale
Artichokes	Red onions	Sweet potatoes
Avocados	Parsley	Spinach
Broccoli	Peppers	Zucchini
Eggplant	Garlic	Green beans
Celery	Onions	Cucumber
Cauliflower	Carrots	Snow peas

Although sweet potatoes are loaded with phytonutrients, they are also slightly higher in sugar. If sweet potatoes appeal to you, I recommend eating a maximum of one serving per day (1 small sweet potato). Remember, white potatoes are to be excluded.

AREN'T AVOCADOS LOADED WITH FAT?

While it is true that avocados are filled with fat, they are filled with the "good fat" called *monounsaturated* fat. You need this fat to lose weight, obtain healthy skin and hair, and to achieve your optimal digestive capacity. In addition, avocados have a high vitamin E content which assists in slowing down aging, and protecting against cancer and heart disease. Due to avocados' higher fat content, they are also significantly higher in calories. The key to gaining avocados' health benefits and avoiding excess calories is to eat them in moderation. One-quarter to one-half an avocado a day in a wrap, on a salad, or in the form of a guacamole dip is both delicious and excellent for your health.

AREN'T CARROTS LOADED WITH SUGAR THAT WILL MAKE ME FAT?

Carrots have received some undeservedly bad press lately due to their higher Glycemic Index (GI) rating (see chapter 4 for more on the GI index). Yet carrots' Glycemic Load, a measurement that quantifies their true carbohydrate content and effect on blood sugar, is significantly lower. In other words, the nutritional value of carrots, which includes an abundant amount of disease-fighting and vision-promoting vitamin A and carotenoids, far outweighs their slight effect on blood sugar levels. In truth, after working with thousands of people, I have never had a client who has become overweight from eating too many carrots. I am not a fan of baby carrots because I don't like their taste. When purchasing carrots for the cleanse, I prefer organic carrots.

Food Fact: A study of more than 125,000 healthcare workers found that just one additional daily serving of fruit or vegetables lowered the risk of heart disease by 4 percent.

Element #7—Drink Eight Glasses of Filtered Water or Herbal Tea Daily

During your five-day cleanse, it is crucial to drink enough water to ensure optimal hydration and a constant flushing out of your system. If you do experience unpleasant symptoms, drinking water will help to diminish them. I recommend starting your day with an 8-ounce glass of filtered water (reverse osmosis or distilled) with fresh-squeezed lemon juice.

I also recommend avoiding all coffee, tea, juice and pop. These items cause dehydration, fluctuation of energy levels and weight gain. Substitute by drinking flavored herbal teas such as peach, blueberry or strawberry for hydration and to help you deal with sugar cravings. In addition, green tea also offers wonderful health benefits such as anti-cancer properties, lowering cholesterol and increasing metabolism. One of several studies on green tea found in the *American Journal of Clinical Nutrition* demonstrated green tea's effectiveness in increasing a process called *thermogenesis*—the body's rate of burning calories. In addition, chemicals in green tea called *polyphenols*, specifically those called catechins, can help prevent obesity by inhibiting the movement of glucose (sugar) into fat cells.

So how much do you need to drink? Research shows that drinking approximately two to three cups of green tea per day is effective at producing the metabolic-boosting and fat-burning effects. However, this amount is too much to be consumed during a cleansing period. Individuals who are caffeine sensitive may feel jittery or experience heart palpitations from this amount. During the five-day cleanse, only drink one cup of green tea as a replacement for your morning coffee. Be sure to drink your green tea with food. Following the cleansing period, drink two to three cups of green tea daily to offer health and weight loss benefits.

I am a huge fan of using matcha in a smoothie or in hot water. Matcha tea is a high-quality green tea that is covered before it is picked to accentuate the color, then stone ground after being picked and before being sealed into small tins.

Matcha can be whisked in hot water in a bowl to make a frothy hot tea or can be added to a smoothie. Among the several health benefits that matcha offers (i.e., alkalinity, boosting metabolism, creating a sense of alertness and prolonged energy, and secreting L-theanine, which helps you to feel calm), matcha also helps to pull toxins into the blood and filter them out of the body. In other words, matcha can help to neutralize free radical damage to assist you with your cleansing process. If you have been "beating up your body" (i.e., through smoking, stress, poor food choices or dehydration) for a long time, too much matcha can make you feel slightly nauseous (you will detox too quickly). Start with 1 tablespoon per day in your smoothie or whisked in hot water. Visit your local tea shop to inquire about their organic matcha options.

WHAT ABOUT COCONUT WATER?

Coconut water is a clear liquid that is low in calories, cholesterol free and contains more potassium than four bananas! It has a sweet, nutty taste and contains easily digested carbohydrates in the form of natural sugars and electrolytes. If drinking coconut water on the cleanse, do not substitute it for plain water—it can be in addition to. Use unsweetened coconut water that contains only 5 calories per ounce and 1 gram of natural sugar. Coconut water is an ideal post-workout drink that helps to rehydrate.

> **Water Facts:** In 37 percent of Americans, the thirst mechanism is so weak that it is often mistaken for hunger. Lack of water is the #1 trigger of daytime fatigue.

Element #8—Consume 1 Tbsp. of Ground Flaxseeds and 2 to 3 Grams of Distilled Fish Oil Daily

During the cleanse, it is very important that you have a minimum of one bowel movement per day to help rid your body of toxic waste. The best method to ensure bowel motility is to introduce a fiber supplement such as ground flaxseeds and fish oils. Ground flaxseeds will act as an "internal dust buster," mopping up unwanted toxic material (metabolic waste). It will also act as a gentle laxative. Fish oils will act as a "conditioner to hair follicles," decreasing intestinal inflammation and creating a positive bowel effect.

Of all the fiber supplements, ground flaxseeds are ultimately the best choice. Flaxseeds contain both soluble and insoluble fiber as well as a special fiber called *mucilage*. Mucilage helps to stabilize blood sugar levels and helps to protect against bowel cancer. In addition, flaxseeds also contain plant chemicals called *lignans* that have anti-cancer, anti-viral, antibacterial and antioxidant properties. In fact, flaxseeds contain 75 to 800 percent more lignans than any other vegetable or grain! Flaxseeds are also a good source of protein (25 grams of protein per every 100 gram of flaxseeds) and omega-3 essential fatty acid. Other flaxseed health properties include:

- Assisting with weight loss
- Buffering excess stomach acid
- Soothing ulcers and irritable bowel disorders
- Lubricating intestinal tract

HOW TO USE FLAXSEEDS

In order to absorb flaxseeds, they have to be ground up or milled. Once ground, add flaxseeds to your morning cereal, salads, juice and protein shakes—or just eat them plain. During the five-day cleanse, take 1 tablespoon of flaxseed every morning with plenty of water to help the fiber flush through your system.

Continue using flaxseeds following the five-day cleanse period for their incredible benefits to your health. Please refer to page 133 for more information on how to pick a fish oil supplement.

Summary of Step 1 — Your Five-Day Cleanse

1. Eliminate all grains.
2. Eliminate all dairy products with the exception of 1 ounce of goat cheese.
3. Eliminate all red meat.
4. Eliminate all white sugar.
5. Take a minimum of three capsules of "friendly bacteria" (probiotic) daily with food.

6. Increase consumption of phytonutrient-rich foods.

7. Drink eight glasses of distilled water or herbal tea daily (no juice, pop, coffee or alcohol).

8. Consume 1 tbsp. of ground flaxseeds and 2–3 grams of fish oil supplements daily.

Five-Day Cleanse — Shopping List

MEATS/PROTEIN SOURCES (3–5 OUNCES PER MEAL)

- Eggs—organic are best
- Lean ground turkey or chicken
- Canned wild Pacific salmon—packed in water, low sodium
- Canned tuna—packed in water, low sodium
- Lean chicken breasts
- Fish—any kind
- Low-sodium canned black beans or chickpeas, or edamame
- Protein powder—brown rice, pea or hemp is suggested

FRUITS (2 SERVINGS PER DAY)

- Avocado
- Frozen mango
- Bananas (small)
- Apples
- Lemons
- Limes
- Berries: blueberries, blackberries or raspberries
- Nectarines, plums, peaches, pears or watermelon

VEGETABLES (EAT AS MUCH AS YOU LIKE!)

- Cauliflower
- Kale
- English cucumber
- Cherry tomatoes (great for munching on, so buy lots)
- Eggplant
- Red peppers
- Organic whole carrots—leave skin on and just rinse well
- Red onions
- Romaine or iceberg lettuce
- Spinach
- Arugula
- Garlic

SPICES, HERBS AND SEASONINGS

- Cinnamon
- Cumin
- Chili powder
- Turmeric
- Tabasco sauce
- Parsley
- Coriander (Cilantro)
- Mint
- Oregano
- Thyme
- Sage
- Dill

DRESSINGS AND SWEETENERS

- Raw, unpasteurized honey
- Apple cider vinegar
- Low-sodium tamari sauce (healthier soy sauce)
- Dijon mustard—regular and grainy

FATS (3 SERVINGS PER DAY)

- Extra virgin olive oil
- Coconut oil
- Organic butter
- Golden or regular ground flaxseeds (also called flax meal)
- Chia seeds
- Raw almonds, pecans or walnuts
- Pistachios, unsalted in shells
- Raw pumpkin seeds, sunflower or sesame seeds
- Tahini
- Nut butters: almond, pecan, walnut or peanut
- Hemp hearts

LIQUIDS/TEAS/HOT DRINKS

- Unsweetened almond milk
- Unsweetened coconut water
- All herbal teas—unlimited (dandelion tea is especially good for detoxification)
- Matcha green tea powder
- Green tea
- Bambu coffee substitute—unlimited

EXTRAS

- Tomato sauce with simple ingredients—low salt and no sugar or preservatives other than ascorbic acid
- Organic chicken broth, low sodium
- Raw cacao nibs

DAIRY

- Goat cheese, herbed or plain (1 ounce per day)

Five-Day Cleanse Meal Plan (serves one)

Each day upon rising, consume:

- 6–8 ounces of warm water with the juice of ½ fresh lemon added
- 1 tablespoon of ground flaxseeds for extra fiber
- Probiotics and fish oil supplements

DAY 1

Breakfast: Apple pancake★
Snack: 1 tablespoon of walnut or almond butter and 1 apple
Lunch: Baked falafels★ with tahini dressing★ and skinny Greek salad★
Snack: Energy in a glass—Combine 1 apple, 1 organic carrot, a handful of spinach and/or kale and 6 ounces of coconut water in a blender. Blend on high and enjoy!
Dinner: Low-carb chicken fajitas★, roasted veggie spread★
Recipes for starred entries (★) are included at end of meal plan.

DAY 2

Breakfast: 2 eggs cooked as you like and 1 small serving of fruit (i.e., ½ cup of berries)
Snack: 2 whole organic carrots with 1 tablespoon of almond butter
Lunch: Mixed greens with goat cheese, walnuts and grilled chicken. Choose desired salad dressing (i.e., balsamic vinaigrette)
Snack: 2 slices of turkey with mustard and red pepper slices
Dinner: 1 cup of turkey chili★, large kale salad with grated carrot, cucumber and cherry tomatoes, with desired dressing

DAY 3

Breakfast: Coconut milk yogurt or goat milk yogurt with blueberries and ground flaxseeds
Snack: ½ cucumber cut in rounds with 1 tablespoon of hummus for dipping
Lunch: 1 cup of turkey chili
Snack: 3 small prunes with 1 almond or walnut stuffed inside
Dinner: Low-carb chicken fajitas★ wrapped in lettuce

DAY 4

Breakfast: Tomato and basil frittata★
Snack: 1 tablespoon of almond or peanut butter and 1 apple or pear
Lunch: Salad with grilled chicken or tuna, cherry tomatoes, pecans and goat cheese
Snack: Roasted veggie spread★, with vegetables to dip (i.e., carrots, celery, cucumber)
Dinner: Walnut-crusted salmon★, arugula salad

DAY 5

Breakfast: Peanut Butter Banana Smoothie with Chocolate Chips★
Snack: 3 prunes with 3 almonds or walnuts tucked inside
Lunch: Skinny Greek salad
Snack: 1 hard-boiled egg and red pepper slices
Dinner: Low-carb nacho salad

Recipes for the Five-Day Cleanse

Please note: All recipes below are appropriate for the five-day cleanse. At the back of the book, the recipes with a smiling face (☺) are appropriate for the five-day cleanse, while those without are for after you have completed the cleanse.

BREAKFAST

APPLE PANCAKE (SERVES ONE)

Ingredients
1 apple, peeled
1–2 eggs
1 tablespoon ground flax meal
½ teaspoon cinnamon
dash of coconut, canola or olive oil

Directions
Grate ½ an apple into a small bowl. Add flax meal, cinnamon, plus 1 or 2 eggs. Mix till incorporated. Drop mixture into a pre-warmed pan with a dash of oil (coconut, canola or olive; melt oil on

low heat and wipe away excess with paper towel). Cook on medium heat till edges look to be setting and then flip and cook through.

TOMATO AND BASIL FRITTATA (SERVES FOUR)

Ingredients

2 teaspoons extra virgin olive oil

1 medium onion, diced

5 basil leaves, chopped

4 large eggs

4 large egg whites

¼ cup grated mozzarella goat cheese

salt and pepper to taste

2 medium vine-ripened tomatoes, cored and thinly sliced crosswise

Directions

Preheat oven to 400 degrees. Heat oil in a 10-inch skillet over medium-low heat. Stir in onion and cook until slightly golden, about 8–10 minutes. In a medium bowl whisk basil, eggs, egg whites, cheese, salt and pepper. Pour the eggs into the skillet, making sure they cover all the onions. Arrange tomatoes in an overlapping pattern on top and season with salt and pepper. When edges begin to set (about 2 minutes) move skillet to oven. Cook about 16–18 minutes. Cut into 4 pieces and serve warm.

"BRING ME TO LIFE" KALE SMOOTHIE (SERVES ONE)

Ingredients

¾ cup almond milk or coconut water, unsweetened

1 cup kale (frozen optional)

¼ frozen banana, roughly chopped

¼ cup frozen mango

2 ice cubes

½ lemon

1 scoop vanilla protein powder or 3 tablespoons hemp hearts

Directions

Add milk alternative, kale, banana, mango and ice cubes to the blender. Squeeze about 1 teaspoon of fresh lemon juice into the blender. Add protein powder or hemp hearts. Blend until all is smooth and enjoy!

PEANUT BUTTER BANANA SMOOTHIE WITH CHOCOLATE CHIPS (SERVES ONE)

Ingredients

¾ cup almond milk or coconut milk, unsweetened

1 tablespoon organic peanut butter

½ frozen banana

1 tablespoon ground flax- or chia seeds

1 tablespoon raw cacao nibs

1 scoop vanilla or chocolate protein powder (brown rice, pea or hemp)

2–3 ice cubes

Directions

Blend all ingredients on high and enjoy!

LUNCH

DAIRY-FREE DELICIOUS CAESAR SALAD (SERVES FOUR)

Ingredients

Dressing
¼ cup tahini

¼ cup water (plus more for thinning)

2 teaspoons freshly grated garlic

2 tablespoons nutritional yeast flakes

2 teaspoons Dijon mustard

¼ teaspoon salt

Salad
2 cups chopped romaine lettuce

2 cups chopped baby arugula

19-ounce (540 ml) can chickpeas, rinsed and drained

1 avocado, peeled and diced

fresh black pepper to taste

Directions
Dressing: Stir together the dressing ingredients in a small bowl, using a fork to blend smooth. Add additional tablespoons of water to thin as needed. Adjust seasoning to taste.

Salad: In a large mixing bowl, toss the greens with the dressing. Add the avocado and chickpeas. Serve with fresh black pepper sprinkled on top.

BAKED FALAFEL LETTUCE WRAPS (SERVES FOUR)

Makes 16 falafels in total—4 falafels per serving

Ingredients

1 19-ounce (540 ml) can chickpeas, rinsed well and drained

1 teaspoon extra virgin olive oil

½ teaspoon ground cumin

1 teaspoon cayenne pepper

1 teaspoon turmeric

1 clove garlic, crushed

1 tablespoon freshly squeezed lemon juice

1 carrot, finely grated

1 tablespoon chopped fresh coriander (if you do not like coriander, use parsley)

pepper to taste

Iceberg lettuce or other large-leaf greens for a grain-free wrap

Directions

Preheat oven to 400 degrees. Cover baking sheet with parchment paper. Place chickpeas in a bowl; add olive oil and mash until smooth. Mix in cumin, cayenne, turmeric, garlic, lemon juice, carrot, coriander and pepper.

Shape into 16 flat, round patties each around 1½ inches across and place on baking sheet. Bake 15–20 minutes total, but flip after 8–10 minutes. Serve warm with lettuce wraps, with a drizzle of tahini dressing.

Please note: Falafels can be frozen once cooked.

TAHINI DRESSING (SERVES SIX TO EIGHT)

Ingredients
⅓ cup tahini

⅓ cup water

¼ cup plus 1 tablespoon fresh lemon juice

2 cloves garlic

dash of salt

Directions
Blend all ingredients until smooth and creamy. Drizzle on falafels or use as a salad dressing.

SKINNY GREEK SALAD (SERVES ONE)

Ingredients

Dressing
2 tablespoons extra virgin olive oil

1 teaspoon lemon juice

1 teaspoon chopped fresh oregano

pinch of sea salt and pepper

Salad
1 English cucumber, finely chopped

1 red pepper, seeded and finely chopped

¼ red onion, finely chopped

3 plum (Roma) tomatoes, finely chopped

½ avocado, chopped into small cubes

3 ounces grilled chicken strips (optional)

Directions

Combine all ingredients in a medium-sized bowl. Mix in dressing and enjoy. Add grilled chicken strips on top if desired for an extra protein punch!

SNACKS

ROASTED VEGGIE SPREAD (SERVES SIX TO EIGHT)

Ingredients

1 medium eggplant, peeled and coarsely chopped into 1-inch cubes

2 red peppers, seeded and coarsely chopped into 1-inch cubes

1 red onion, peeled and coarsely chopped

2 cloves garlic, peeled

1 tablespoon extra virgin olive oil

pinch of sea salt and ground black pepper

1 tablespoon tomato paste

Directions

Preheat oven to 400 degrees. Combine chopped eggplant, peppers, onion and garlic in a bowl and toss with olive oil and salt and pepper. Spread on a baking sheet and roast for 45 minutes, tossing once halfway through baking. Add tomato paste and cool slightly then place veggies in a food processor and pulse 3 or 4 times. Mixture should have a slightly chunky texture.

MASHED CAULIFLOWER (SERVES TWO)

Ingredients

1 head of cauliflower, chopped

1 clove garlic, peeled

salt and pepper

1 tablespoon butter

Directions

Roast or steam cauliflower with garlic for 7–10 minutes (until cauliflower is soft). Add salt and pepper to taste. Drain and mash with fork or hand mixer, add butter and continue mashing until the cauliflower has a creamy and smooth consistency.

DINNER

WALNUT-CRUSTED SALMON (SERVES FOUR)

Ingredients

1 cup chopped walnuts

2 tablespoons ground flaxseeds

2 tablespoons grated lemon rind

1 tablespoon extra virgin olive oil

1 teaspoon dried or fresh dill

salt and pepper to taste

4 salmon fillets, skin on

2 teaspoons Dijon mustard

lemon juice

Directions

In food processor, blend walnuts, flaxseeds, lemon rind, oil, dill, salt and pepper using pulsing action until crumbly (mixture should slightly stick together) and set aside. Place salmon fillets skin-side down and brush tops with mustard. Divide crust mixture evenly among the fillets and press onto the mustard, on both sides of the fillet. Allow to sit in fridge for at least 15 minutes and up to 2 hours. Bake in 350-degree oven for about 15 minutes or until salmon flakes when touched with a fork. Drizzle with lemon juice.

TURKEY CHILI (SERVES SIX)

Ingredients
1 pound lean ground chicken or turkey

1 onion, coarsely chopped

2 large cloves garlic, minced

1 teaspoon chili powder

1 teaspoon ground cumin

½ teaspoon oregano

pinch of salt and pepper

1 19-ounce (540 ml) can low-sodium kidney or black beans, rinsed and drained

4 fresh plum tomatoes, chopped

1 red pepper, chopped into chunks

1 cup fresh tomato pasta sauce

Directions
Cook ground chicken/turkey till brown in heavy saucepan or wok (approximately 5 minutes), then pour off any excess fat. Add onions, garlic, chili, cumin, oregano, salt and pepper and stir over low heat until onions are tender. Stir in kidney beans (or black beans), plum tomatoes, red pepper and tomato sauce and bring to a boil. Reduce heat and simmer for 20 minutes.

LOW-CARB CHICKEN FAJITAS (SERVES FOUR)

Ingredients

16 ounces boneless, skinless chicken breasts

3 tablespoons lime juice

1 teaspoon ground cumin

1 teaspoon garlic powder

pinch of chili powder to taste

pinch of salt and pepper to taste

1 medium onion, sliced

1 red pepper, cut into strips

1 green or yellow pepper, cut into strips

2 teaspoons extra virgin olive oil

iceberg lettuce or other large-leaf greens for a grain-free wrap

½ cup salsa (optional)

4 ounces goat cheese (optional)

Directions

Marinate chicken breasts in lime juice for 1 hour, then season with cumin, garlic powder, chili powder, salt and pepper. Season onion and peppers with salt and pepper and toss with olive oil. Cook in skillet over medium heat for approximately 15 minutes. Grill chicken until cooked through, about 8 minutes on each side. Transfer to a cutting board when done and cut into strips. Once cooked, combine with cooked onion and peppers. Rip lettuce leaves into "wrap-like" pieces and add chicken and vegetables. Top with salsa and/or goat cheese if desired.

CHIPLESS NACHOLESS SALAD (SERVES TWO)

Ingredients

1½ cups shredded iceberg lettuce

½ pound ground chicken, cooked

½ cup sliced black olives

½ cup chopped tomatoes

¼ cup chopped green onions

½ cup shredded goat cheese

Directions

On a baking pan lined with tinfoil, spread a bed of shredded lettuce. Evenly distribute cooked ground chicken, olives, chopped tomatoes, green onions and any additional toppings (try red peppers, green peppers or hot peppers). Sprinkle with cheese. Heat oven to 350 degrees and broil for 3 minutes or until cheese is bubbling. Remove immediately and serve.

More Five-Day Cleanse Meal Options (serve one)

BREAKFAST OPTIONS

1. **Strawberry banana smoothie**
   Combine ½ banana, 1 scoop of protein powder, ¼ cup of unsweetened almond milk, ¼ cup of water, ¼ cup of frozen or fresh strawberries, 1 tbsp. of flaxseed oil. Blend well.

2. **Mango, blueberry banana shake**

   Combine ½ banana, 3 large slices of mango, ½ cup
   of blueberries, ½ cup of unsweetened almond milk,
   1 scoop of protein powder, ½ cup of water, 1 tbsp. of
   flaxseed oil. Blend well.

3. **Cheesy scrambled eggs with mushrooms**

   1 tsp. of butter, 4 pasteurized egg whites, 1 whole egg,
   ¼ cup of mushrooms and 1 ounce of goat cheese.
   Add butter to frying pan and cook all ingredients over
   medium heat.

4. Fresh fruit salad and hard-boiled egg, ½ cup of strawberries, melon cubes and blueberries.

5. Poached egg (1), ½ grapefruit, ½ handful of almonds.

LUNCH OPTIONS

1. **Tuna salad**

   4 ounces of tuna, 2 cups of mixed greens, sliced
   tomato and onion, 2 tbsp. of light dressing, e.g., rasp-
   berry vinaigrette.

2. **Veggie chili or dairy-free soup** (e.g., pea soup,
   lentil soup, tomato soup) with salad and vinaigrette
   or olive oil dressing.

3. **Chicken breast on green salad**

   3-ounce chicken breast, 2 cups of mixed greens with
   flaxseed oil dressing (see recipe on page 127).

4. **Grilled wild salmon on spinach salad**

   4-ounce wild salmon fillet, 2 cups baby spinach, ⅓
   cup sliced mushrooms, ½ cup mandarin oranges, 2
   tbsp. of light balsamic vinaigrette dressing.

5. **Asian omelet**

   1 whole egg, 4 egg whites, 1 cup fresh bean sprouts,
   diced onions, basil, dash of soy sauce, 1 tsp. butter.

DINNER OPTIONS

1. **Chicken teriyaki stir-fry**
   3-ounce boneless, skinless chicken breast with 1½ cups mix of chopped zucchini, mushrooms, red pepper, and onion. Lightly stir-fry with teriyaki sauce.

2. **3-ounce wild salmon fillet** (broiled) with asparagus and 1 small sweet potato.

3. **Egg white omelet with black beans**
   4 pasteurized egg whites, 1 whole egg, ¼ cup black beans, diced onion and red pepper, 1 tsp. butter.

4. **Veggie patty** (1, any brand) and 1 cup steamed vegetables of your choice (i.e., broccoli, spinach, carrots, cauliflower) with lemon juice.

5. **Grilled chicken salad with walnuts**
   2 cups chopped romaine lettuce, 2-ounce grilled skinless chicken breast strips, 2 tbsp. crushed walnuts, 2 tbsp. vinaigrette dressing.

SNACK OPTIONS

1. Hummus (chickpea dip) and carrots
2. Sliced strawberries, bananas and unsweetened almond milk with cinnamon and crushed walnuts
3. Natural nut butter on celery
4. Coconut yogurt with fruit
5. Baked apples

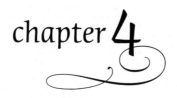

chapter 4

STEP 2—NOURISH

"The doctor of the future will give no medicine, but will interest his patients in the care of the human body, in diet, and in the cause and prevention of disease."

—THOMAS EDISON

*N*ow that you have finished your five-day cleanse, it is time to move onto steps 2, 3 and 4. Step 2 is called the nourish step as it will flood your system with the critical nutrients necessary to climb to your highest level of health. What exactly do I mean by this? By following the nutritional recommendations outlined in step 2, the delicious food choices you consume will nourish your body and will be the strongest weapon against potential beauty robbers and future illness or disease. By following the unique Pick-3 System of eating, your body will soon shed any cobwebs of ill health or excess weight and will enter the "health groove" for good. As you will soon discover, you will not have to cut calories or feel restricted in your food choices. The right type and amount of grains, fruits, vegetables, lean meats and fish, nuts and seeds are all recommended and encouraged. The nourish step is not a program that you go off of in a week or two. There are no points to count, shakes to drink or meals to skip. Once you understand the principles, you will be able to apply them to your eating habits for a lifetime, reaping the continual satisfaction of energetic living and optimal health.

The four elements involved in the nourish step are:

1. Forget low carb—eat slow carb!
2. Consume lean proteins at every meal or snack.
3. Eat essential fats.
4. Follow the Pick-3 System of eating—it keeps your metabolism revved and weight down!

Element #1 — Forget Low Carb — Eat Slow Carb!

"Everything that exceeds the bounds of moderation has an unstable foundation."

—Lucius Seneca

Carbohydrates provide 4 calories per gram.

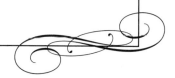

Every decade or so, the nutritional world undergoes a dieting craze or a fad way of eating which catches on. In the 1980s, low-fat diets were the latest craze with low-fat food products popping up on every grocery shelf. The results of eating low fat were fairly grim with people gaining more and more weight, all the while eating low-fat foods. Why did it fail so miserably? Fat is one of the main components that makes food taste good. Without fat, food does not have the same appeal or texture. If low-fat products did not have a little extra "something" added to enhance taste, no one would buy them as they would taste terrible. In order to add flavor to a product labeled "low fat" and to tempt the palate of potential consumers, food manufacturers typically add sugar or artificial sweeteners to low-fat products—and lots of it! As you will discover in the section below on eating slow carbohydrates, with the addition of sugar or artificial sweeteners, weight gain and immune system suppression is inevitable—which ultimately resulted in failure of the low-fat craze.

Food Fact: In the height of the low-carb craze that has recently passed, some 26 million Americans were on a hardcore low-carb diet and 70 million more limit their carb intake.

Currently, in the year 2014, we are on the tail end of yet another nutritional craze—the low-carbohydrate craze. Atkins, the South Beach diet and the Paleo diet are just a few of the several low-carbohydrate programs that are enormously popular. In an attempt to lose weight, people are going extremely "hard core low-carb" and were cutting out this precious component of their diets completely. Although it is true that certain carbohydrates are best left for occasional indulgences, as you will see, cutting out carbohydrates completely can result in a wide range of health problems such as:

- Constipation due to lack of fiber
- An overly acidic system
- Ingestion of too many saturated fats, which can lead to hardening of the arteries, heart disease and high blood pressure
- Extreme stress on the kidneys
- Yo-yo dieting, which makes every future attempt at losing weight harder and harder

Food Fact: 1,558 low-carb products have hit stores since 2002.

When considering your food options, keep in mind that there are three types of foods called *macronutrients* that are essential to health and should be included in every diet: 1) carbohydrates, 2) proteins and 3) fats. Let's examine carbohydrates first.

Carbohydrates are found in fruits, vegetables, legumes and grains such as cereal, breads, pasta and rice and are the body's main source of fuel. In order to eat carbohydrates effectively to optimize digestion, lose or maintain your body weight, and look and feel your best, the key is to consume mostly slow carbohydrates.

What Are Slow Carbs?

Slow carbohydrates are found in vegetables, most fruits, whole grain breads and legumes. They are the key to maintaining a constant energy source without negative consequences such as weight gain, lack of energy, mood fluctuation or mental fogginess. Slow carbohydrates are the ticket to internal health, weight loss and external beauty and vigor. To understand how they work, let's examine how the body utilizes carbohydrates.

The body breaks down carbohydrates into sugar called *glucose* to be used as the primary source of fuel for the body. Glucose is then transferred into the cells and used as an energy source. In fact, certain areas of the body such as the brain and red blood cells rely exclusively on glucose as fuel. Other parts of the body can use other sources of fuel such as fat or protein, but none burn as efficiently and cleanly as carbohydrates.

The key to eating the right type of carbohydrates lies in understanding the intricate relationship between blood glucose levels and insulin. Insulin is a hormone secreted from the pancreas in response to elevated blood glucose levels. Blood glucose and insulin are in constant communication. Of insulin's many roles in the body, one is to transport glucose into the cells to be used as fuel. The membrane (external barrier) of all cells has "gates" that open up to allow the glucose into the cell to be absorbed. The process works like this:

1. Blood glucose levels are elevated by eating a specific food, for instance, a piece of bread.
2. The pancreas responds to the elevation of blood glucose by secreting insulin.
3. Insulin opens up the gates of cells to allow glucose to enter.
4. The gates of the cell open, and glucose gets absorbed into the cells.
5. Blood glucose levels are normalized.

Figure 4.1: Carbohydrates, Glucose and Insulin Relationship

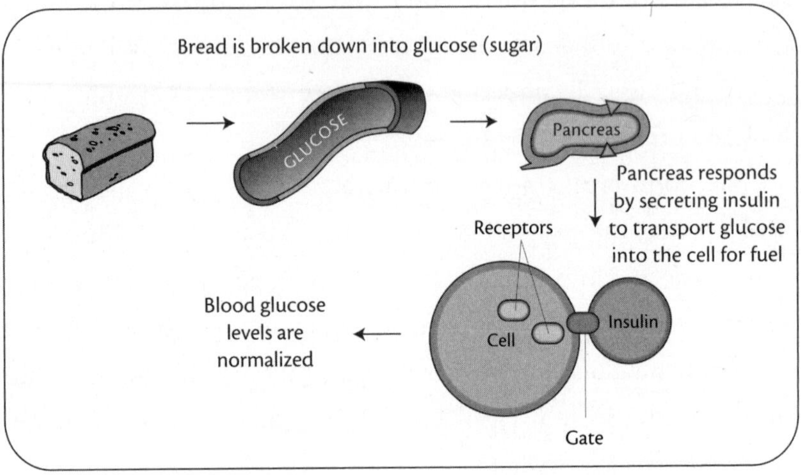

So why all the fuss about carbohydrates, weight gain and low-carb foods? Because certain foods such as refined flour and sugar products cause the oversecretion of the hormone insulin. When insulin is oversecreted, blood sugar levels drop too low and a "crash" occurs, sending the poor individual into a state of hypoglycemia (low blood sugar). This results in fatigue, moodiness, hunger, mental fogginess and cravings for more carbohydrates. To make matters worse, excess insulin secretion triggers glucose to be stored as excess fat! In other words, the more refined foods you eat, the more insulin you will secrete. In turn, you will experience more cravings, mood and energy fluctuations throughout the day and you will gain more weight.

Foods that tend to be an oversecretor of insulin include:

- White sugary foods—i.e., candy, pop, cookies, cakes, muffins
- White rice

- White pasta
- White potatoes—baked and mashed
- White bread
- Raisins and dates
- Refined cereal—i.e., Corn Flakes, rice cereals

It is important to remember that insulin secretion is not the enemy. In fact, a normal secretion of insulin as a result of eating a specific food is expected and desired, while an oversecretion of insulin is not. Too much insulin secretion can be the underlying cause of many health problems. These include:

- Excess weight gain
- Fluctuation in mood and energy levels
- Cravings
- Fatigue
- Poor blood sugar control leading to Type II diabetes
- Syndrome X (a.k.a. metabolic syndrome)
- Cardiovascular disease

The good news is there is a way to eat the foods you love, all the while controlling your blood sugar and insulin levels. The key in determining which foods cause an oversecretion of insulin and which do not is to refer to the Glycemic Index (GI) and Glycemic Load (GL). (For more information, see the appendix.) The Glycemic Index is a tool that measures the specific rate of a food item into the bloodstream. The faster the speed of entry, the more insulin will be secreted. For ranking purposes, the Glycemic Index is divided into three categories: low, medium and high. Food is categorized from a scale of 0 to 100 depending on its effect on blood sugar levels. On the Glycemic Index scale, the highest measurement is for glucose which is ranked 100. For the most part, foods that are lowest on the Glycemic Index have the slowest rate of entry into the bloodstream and therefore have the lowest insulin response. The categories are:

- Low—up to 55
- Medium—56 to 70
- High—over 70

To gain all the benefits of eating carbohydrates while avoiding excess insulin secretion, it is important to stick to low- to medium-ranked carbohydrates. For the most part, all vegetables (with the exception of white potatoes), most fruits (with the exception of dates, raisins and lychee fruit), whole grains and beans are ranked fairly low on the Glycemic Index. Processed foods such as white bread, white flour, cereals, pretzels, muffins, candy, pop and breakfast bars are ranked higher. Consider the following examples.

High GI Foods — Fast Carbs

Fast carbohydrates = ↑ insulin = excess weight gain = cravings, fatigue, moodiness

- White plain baguette—95
- White flour—70
- Wonder enriched white bread—77
- English muffin—77
- Kellogg's Corn Flakes—80
- White boiled rice—72

- Puffed rice cakes—82
- Raisins—64
- Dates—103
- Lychee fruit—79
- Brown rice pasta—92
- Strawberry fruit bar—91
- Jelly beans—80
- Baked potato—85
- Instant mashed potatoes—85

Low GI Foods — Slow Carbs

Slow carbohydrates = normal insulin secretion = weight loss or maintenance of weight = optimal energy

- All-Bran cereal—30
- Coarse white kernel bread—41
- Spelt multigrain bread—54
- Long grain boiled rice—41
- Low-fat fruit yogurt—31
- Grapes—46
- Apple—34
- Orange—42
- Plum—39
- Strawberries—40
- Black-eyed beans—33
- Chickpeas—31
- Navy beans—38
- Lentils—29
- Protein enriched spaghetti—27
- Sweet potato—61
- Green peas—48

Health Tip: To keep your weight down, do not eat grains past 4 p.m.

There are several factors that can affect the GI of a food:

1. Fiber
2. Protein
3. Fat
4. Cooking
5. Processing

Fiber, protein and fat act as a brake to lower Glycemic Index ratings. This is why vegetables and fruits which are higher in fiber and protein-enriched spaghetti have a lower GI rating. This is also why the candy M&Ms have a lower GI rating of 41—they are loaded with fat! The fact that a highly nutritious orange (GI 40) and M&Ms have almost the same GI rating highlights an important point. The Glycemic Index rating is an effective tool for measuring only the speed of entry of a food item into the bloodstream—*not* the health value of a food.

The World Health Organization estimates that low intake of fruits and vegetables causes 19 percent of gastrointestinal cancer, 31 percent of ischemic heart disease and 11 percent of strokes.

Food Fact: Undercooking your pasta—making it "el dente"—will lower the GI value, resulting in less insulin secretion.

The processing and cooking of a food source also affect GI ratings by knocking out the amount of fiber that was once in a whole grain item. For example, a refined piece of white bread has a high GI rating and whole grain coarse kernel bread has a low GI rating. The processing and refining of flours for fluffier breads, pastas and pastries is one of the major contributors to the obesity epidemic we are currently experiencing. The refining process pulverizes whole grain foods into refined flours thereby eliminating the fiber content (the brake), enabling the flour to rush into the bloodstream very rapidly. As you will see in the Pick-3 System of eating, simply combining your carbohydrates with the proper fat and protein slows down this process, allowing the body to maintain hormonal balance, lose weight and function at an optimal state of health and wellness.

Food Fact: As a general rule, tropical fruits like bananas and pineapples are rated higher on the Glycemic Index, while more temperate fruits such as berries, cherries, pears and apples are rated lower on the Glycemic Index.

Due to the occasional inaccuracies of the Glycemic Index, there is an additional tool used which is designed to measure blood sugar response to specific foods, called the Glycemic Load. The Glycemic Load tells you how much sugar is in the food, rather than just how high it raises blood sugar levels. In other words, it considers a food's Glycemic Index as well as the amount of carbohydrates per serving. The calculation of the Glycemic Load is the Glycemic Index divided by 100 and multiplied by its available carbohydrate content. The values are:

- High—20
- Medium—11 to 19
- Low—10 and under

Let's compare the Glycemic Load of two different food items. Carrots have received some undeserved bad press recently due to their sugar content and high Glycemic Index rating of 71. Yet, on closer examination, carrots only have 4 grams of carbohydrates in total. To determine the Glycemic Load of carrots, the calculation is:

$$71 \times 0.04 = 2.84 \text{ GL}$$

Therefore, carrots have a low Glycemic Load rating and will not oversecrete the hormone insulin. As mentioned, I have never had a patient become obese or suffer from ill health from eating too many carrots! Now let's take the example of 1 cup of cooked, white pasta that also has a Glycemic Index rating of 71, but contains 40 grams of carbohydrate. The calculation is:

$$71 \times 0.40 = 28.4 \text{ GL}$$

You can see that pasta has a high Glycemic Load because it is so dense in carbohydrates.

The following food tips will help you stick to foods that rank low on the Glycemic Index and Glycemic Load:

- Eat a wide variety of non-starchy vegetables.
- Replace refined foods with whole grain products, e.g., whole grain bread instead of white bread.
- Eat fruits and starchy vegetables with high-protein

or high-fiber foods, e.g., add flaxseeds or protein powder to your meal or snack. See the Pick-3 System of eating (page 109) for more examples.

- Use healthy fats found in nuts, seeds, grains, fish and liquid oils (olive, canola, soybean, etc.).

> Turn to your fridge for a makeover! Vegetables that are especially good for a wrinkle-free complexion include garlic, broccoli, stawberries, blueberries and dark leafy greens.

Element #2 — Consume Lean Proteins at Every Meal or Snack

Proteins are the second category of macronutrients that are an equally necessary part of every diet. In terms of protein consumption, there are usually two camps. Either people follow the traditional and outdated food pyramid that recommends too little protein and too many carbohydrates in the form of bread, cereal and pasta or they follow a high-protein diet in an attempt to lose weight and are eating an excessive amount of the wrong types of proteins. Both of these approaches have cracks and can rob internal health and upset metabolism. Eating the wrong type of protein or consuming too little or too much can erode external beauty and internal health and lead to numerous health problems such as excess weight gain, inflammation, poor complexion, dry skin, fatigue and premature aging. The key to eating protein properly is to consume the right source of lean protein at each and every meal or snack.

> Protein provides 4 calories per gram.

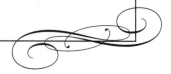

Proteins serve many functions in the body such as maintaining proper growth and repair of muscles and tissues; manufacturing hormones, antibodies and enzymes; and preserving the proper acid-alkali balance in the body. In addition, proteins facilitate the release of the hormone *glucagon*, which has an opposing effect to insulin. This is why adding protein to a meal immediately lowers the secretion of insulin, thereby causing less weight gain. Unfortunately, due to the surge in high-protein diets, many people were eating the wrong type of protein in excess in an attempt to lose weight. Red meats such as steak, bacon, ribs, cold cuts and hamburgers are typically loaded with artery-clogging and inflammatory saturated fats. These types of fats have been linked with a multitude of disease processes including heart disease, stroke, high blood pressure, cancer and hormonal disturbances in both men and women.

Lean proteins are the type of proteins you want to include in your daily diet. These include:

- Lean turkey or chicken breast
- Fish such as wild salmon, tuna (use sparingly and use light, not white, tuna), sole, cod, clams, oysters, mackerel, haddock, halibut, crab, lobster, sardines, sea bass, shrimp, trout (freshwater), tilapia and scallops
- Egg whites and omega-3 eggs
- Low-fat yogurt
- Skim milk
- Low-fat cottage cheese or other low-fat cheeses
- Goat cheese
- Protein powder
- Tofu: veggie burgers, imitation ground beef, seasoned firm tofu in a stir-fry
- Soy cheese

- Soy milk
- Tempeh (soybean cake with a smoky, nutty flavor. It can be marinated or grilled and added to stir-fries, casseroles or chili.)
- Occasional lean beef or pork

> To reduce the amount of mercury that you ingest with tuna, use canned chunk light tuna instead of canned white albacore tuna.

SAMPLE SERVING SIZES OF PROTEIN

The palm of your hand, minus your thumb and fingers, or a deck of cards equals a 3-ounce serving of fish or meat.

- 1 scoop of protein powder = 25 grams of protein
- 4 ounces of chicken or fish = 28 grams of protein
- 3 ounces of sirloin steak = 25 grams of protein
- ½ cup of egg whites = 13 grams of protein
- 1 ounce of low-fat cheese = 7 grams of protein
- 1 cup of lima beans = 15 grams of protein
- 4 ounces of firm tofu = 10 grams of protein

On average, women require 70–90 grams of protein per day and men require 100–120 grams of protein per day. To properly include proteins in your diet, refer to the Pick-3 System of eating. This system eliminates measuring or weighing individual food items.

Element #3 — Eat Essential Fats

> Fat provides 9 calories per gram, more than twice the number of calories provided by carbohydrates or protein.

Fat is the third type of macronutrient the body relies on to run smoothly. There are "good" fats and "bad" fats. Certain types of fats are so critical to the functioning of our system that without them, our health and beauty would instantly suffer. In fact, 60 percent of our brain is comprised of fat! The "good" type of fat is also the key factor in keeping digestion running smoothly, inflammation at bay, a wrinkle-free complexion and smooth skin, shiny hair and strong nails. To top it off—you actually need to eat the good type of fat to lose weight!

Do not feel badly if you are confused about how to eat fat. Fats can be confusing to understand as there is such a wide variety in selecting and deciphering the "good" from the "bad." In order to understand the various types of fats available, I have broken them into 5 categories:

1. Trans fatty acids—the "very bad" fats
2. Saturated fats—the "bad" fats
3. Polyunsaturated fats—the "so-so" fats
4. Monounsaturated fats—the "good" fats
5. Essential fats—the "very good" fats

TRANS FATTY ACIDS (TFAS)

Trans fats are the "very bad" fats found in numerous foods on our grocery store shelves such as commercially packaged cookies and crackers, commercially fried food such as French fries, micro-waved popcorn, vegetable shortening and some margarines. Trans fatty acids are the artificial fats that occur when technologists alter the chemical structure of a polyunsaturated fat, i.e., a vegetable oil from a round shape to a straight chain. This process is called *hydrogenation* and involves flooding a polyunsaturated fat with an abundant amount of hydrogen atoms at a high temperature. So what's the big deal about changing the shape of a little fat molecule? Unfortunately, these synthetic fats are known to promote the build-up of plaque in arteries, increase cholesterol levels, promote cancer by causing dangerous defects in cell membranes and increase the risk of cardiovascular disease. In addition, due to their shape, trans fatty acids are extremely difficult for the body to get rid of. According to Dr. Andrew Weil, author of *Eating Well for Optimum Health* (HarperCollins, 2001):

> *It is clear that trans-fatty acids are bad for hearts and arteries. They drive up production of cholesterol like saturated fats and promote atherosclerosis, undoing any benefits that oils might have provided. I am certain that TFAs will eventually be found to be detrimental to health in many other ways as a result of their effects on membrane and hormone function. I believe they promote the development of cancer and obstruct immunity and healing. Therefore, I make a scrupulous attempt to keep them out of the diet, and I urge you to do the same. In practice, that means avoiding margarine, vegetable shortening, and all kinds of products made with them or partially hydrogenated oils of any kind.*

So, how do you identify a food product that contains dangerous trans fatty acids? The good news is that as of January 2006, food manufacturers are required to list the amount of trans fatty acids that are present in their products. This labeling restriction is of the utmost importance since the Food and Drug Administration (FDA) estimates that 2,100 to 5,600 lives are lost each year, and 6,300 to 17,100 cases of fatal and non-fatal coronary heart disease occur each year, because of the lack of trans fat labeling. According to regulation, trans fats must appear on the Nutrition Facts panel. The amount of trans fats per serving of food will appear under the Total Fat section of the label. However, under the FDA regulations, if a product contains less than 0.5 grams of trans fat, it may declared as zero. This should be kept in mind if you eat 3–4 servings of an item. You could be eating as much as 2 grams of trans fat!

In addition to checking labels, if you see the words "hydrogenated" or "partially hydrogenated" oils or fat, then move on. The food in question contains TFAs. If a label still does not yet list the amount of TFAs, you can determine this value on your own. Simply add up the values for saturated, polyunsaturated and monounsaturated fats. If the number is less than the "total fats" shown on the label, the unaccounted fat is derived from trans fat.

Table 4.1: Trans Fats Found in Various Food Products

Product	Common serving size	Total fat grams	Saturated fat grams	Trans fat grams
French fries	Medium (147 grams)	27	7	8
Butter	1 tbsp.	11	7	0
Margarine stick	1 tbsp.	11	2	3
Shortening	1 tbsp.	13	3.5	4
Donut	1	18	4.5	5
Candy bar	1 (40 grams)	10	4	3
Pound cake	1 slice	16	3.5	4.5

In April 2004, the FDA Food Advisory Committee voted in favor of recommending that trans fatty acid intake levels be reduced to "less than 1 percent of energy" or "2 grams of a 2000-calorie diet."

SATURATED FATS

These "bad" fats are usually solid or almost solid at room temperature. They are found in animal products such as butter, cheese,
whole milk, ice cream, cream, and fatty meats. They are also found
in some vegetable oils—palm and palm kernel oils. I refer to saturated fats as the "bad fats" because they make the body produce
more cholesterol, which raises blood cholesterol levels. Excessive
consumption of saturated fats can raise the level of the bad cholesterol known as *low-density lipoprotein* (LDL). High LDL levels (above
160 mg/dL) increase heart disease risk because they keep cholesterol in blood circulation and carry it to the arteries to be deposited.
In addition to raising LDL levels, eating too many of the wrong
fats such as saturated and trans fatty acids increases inflammation.
According to a study appearing in the *American Journal of Clinical
Nutrition*, within an hour of eating a fatty meal, participants experienced increases in inflammatory proteins associated with heart
disease. Levels remained elevated for as long as three to four hours
after the meal.

When looking at a food label, pay very close attention to the
percentage of saturated fat and avoid or limit any foods that are high
in this (over 20% saturated fat). Saturated fats should be kept to 5
percent or less of total dietary fat intake.

Table 4.2: LDL Cholesterol Levels

Less than 100 mg/dL	Optimal
100 to 129 mg/dL	Near Optimal/Above Optimal
130 to 159 mg/dL	Borderline High
160 to 189 mg/dL	High
190 mg/dL and above	Very High

Food Fact: Eating plenty of nuts and sunflower seeds is recommended for their protein, essential fat and vitamin C and E content. Vitamin C and E will help keep skin healthy by retaining more elasticity and resiliency. This ultimately results in fewer wrinkles and lines!

POLYUNSATURATED FAT

Polyunsaturated fat is found in vegetable oils made from safflowers, corn, sunflowers and soybeans. This type of fat remains liquid at room temperature. Although polyunsaturated fat lowers the level of the bad cholesterol lipid known as low-density lipoprotein (LDL), it is also believed to lower the *good* cholesterol lipid, known as high-density lipoprotein (HDL). As you will discover in the following chapter, eating too many omega-6 polyunsaturated fats in the form of refined vegetable oils decreases the amount of a necessary fat called omega-3.

Liposuction reduces the number of fat cells in the body, but it does not decrease the amount of fat that is left in the remaining fat cells.

MONOUNSATURATED FATS

One of the healthiest diets in the world is the Mediterranean diet. Part of the reason that this diet is deemed so "heart healthy" is because it is filled with monounsaturated fats. These "good fats" are found in olive, canola and peanut oils, and in avocados. These fats appear to lower "bad cholesterol" (LDL) and have minimal or no effect on the "good cholesterol" (HDL). Olive oil contains the highest amount of monounsaturated fats of all the edible oils. The best type of olive oil is labeled "extra virgin," made from the first pressing of the olives. This oil is very flavorful and can be used for cooking or in salad dressings. All oils should be stored in dark, cool places.

ESSENTIAL FATS

Essential fats are members of the polyunsaturated fat family. They are called essential fatty acids because they are vital for health and cannot be produced by the body. Every living cell in the body needs essential fatty acids to rebuild and produce new cells. There are two basic categories of essential fatty acids:

1. Omega-3 fatty acids called alpha-linolenic acid
2. Omega-6 fatty acids called linoleic acid

Although a certain amount of omega-6 and omega-3 is necessary in the diet, a problem arises when too many omega-6 fats are consumed. The balance of omega-6 to omega-3 is very important and has a teeter-totter effect. In other words, if an individual has too much of one kind, she will become deficient in the other. Too many polyunsaturated fats in the form of processed vegetable oils creates an imbalance in the ratio of omega-6 essential fatty acids to omega-3 essential fatty acids. Unfortunately, many refined and processed products found on our grocery store shelves are loaded with refined vegetable oils.

Most North Americans are chronically deficient in omega-3 essential fats. Allergies, eczema, inflammatory conditions (i.e., arthritis, colitis), constipation, attention deficit disorder (ADD), dry skin and premature aging have all been linked to a deficiency of this precious fat. While the ideal ratio of omega-6 to omega-3 fat is approximately

1:1, due to the overconsumption of safflower and sunflower oils, and the increase in consumption of processed foods, the average ratio ranges between 20:1 and 30:1.

Figure 4.2: Omega-3:Omega-6 Ratios

Typical North American Ratio   Ideal Ratio

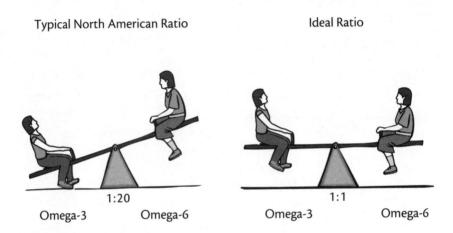

1:20		1:1	
Omega-3	Omega-6	Omega-3	Omega-6

Optimal omega-3 food sources are flaxseed oil, omega-3 eggs, deepwater fish and fish oil, walnuts and walnut oil, and soybeans. Optimal sources of omega-6 are those found in raw nuts, seeds, legumes, borage oil, grapeseed oil and primrose oil. Chapter 5 reviews in detail how to incorporate the proper omega-3 fat into your daily diet for the best skin, hair and weight results.

> The typical American diet tends to contain 11 to 30 times more omega-6 fatty acids than omega-3 fatty acids. Many researchers believe this imbalance is a significant factor in the rising rate of inflammatory disorders.

Element #4 — Follow the Pick-3 System of Eating for Weight Loss

Currently, there are several diet programs on the market that recommend various amounts and types of foods to eat. From extreme low-calorie to crazy high-protein approaches, there is no shortage of literature to read on how to lose weight. As you will soon discover, I strongly believe every macronutrient—protein, fat and carbohydrate—has its place in the diet. However, the right type, combination and amount is critical to your weight loss success. My advice is to ask yourself the following question prior to starting any weight loss program: "Can I see myself following a version of this program for five years or longer?" If the answer is no, it is highly likely that the program is not based in science, cannot be followed long term and will likely result in weight loss that is temporary. The only thing the body dislikes more than being overweight is gaining and losing weight repeatedly—it is time to stop all yo-yo "quick fix" dieting approaches.

This is where following the Pick-3 System of eating comes in. Over the years, I have had the pleasure and experience of working with thousands of clients who wanted and needed to lose weight. To view some of the amazing transformations, visit www.shulmanweightloss.com. I have been able to clearly identify which approaches work, and which do not. It doesn't matter if someone needs to lose 5 or 100 pounds; the same principles apply. I have found that having people follow tricky and time-consuming approaches such as counting points or grams of food or weighing their food ultimately results in failure. Food is meant to be easy and enjoyed. Ultimately, by following the latest diet "schtick," motivation will wane, the program will become tired sooner rather than later, resulting in one more failed attempt to add to the pile. I strongly believe you should not have to keep going on and off an eating program. The method of eating you choose should work for life.

In answer to this need for a system of eating that works long term, motivates and helps women to achieve their weight and beauty goals from the inside out, I have designed the Pick-3 System of eating for weight loss. This system offers enough variety and flexibility that it can be followed for a lifetime. It also ensures that you are taking in all the proper macronutrients to keep your metabolism revved, your energy up and your immune system strong. By eating in this way, you will also be sure to get the proper *phytochemicals* (plant chemicals) in your diet and enough of the "good fats" that will keep your skin, hair and nails looking their best.

Although you do not need to count calories, grams of foods or points that relate to specific foods, the overall, optimal breakdown of food that you will be eating by following the Pick-3 System is:

- 40 percent of calories derived from slow carbo-hydrates
- 30 percent of calories derived from lean proteins
- 30 percent of calories derived from essential fats

So how does the Pick-3 System of eating work? By picking a food source from each of the three columns outlined in table 4.3 at every meal or snack, you are guaranteed to eat a combination of food that does not surge blood sugar levels and, in turn, ensures you lose weight. Even better, because we all have a variety of dietary likes and dislikes, the Pick-3 System of eating is diverse and flexible enough to fit any-one's palate. Instead of tediously counting calories or measuring grams, simply pick a food item from each food column, combine and enjoy!

Table 4.3: The Pick-3 System of Eating

Pick 1—Slow Carbohydrates	Pick 2—Lean Proteins	Pick 3—Essential Fats
Any vegetable, with the exception of white potatoes. Examples are: broccoli cauliflower kale spinach carrots bok choy onions garlic romaine lettuce green beans red and/or green cabbage sweet potatoes yams, zucchini tomatoes, peppers collard greens, eggplant	Meat and meat alternatives. These include skinless turkey, chicken, lamb, salmon, cod, herring, sardines, light tuna, sole, cod, mackerel, haddock, crab, lobster, sardines, sea bass, shrimp, trout and scallops, egg whites and omega-3 eggs, soy products (miso, tempeh, tofu, fortified soy milk, tofu cheese), occasional extra lean beef or pork. • 4–6 ounces per serving	Raw almonds or walnuts, raw sunflower seeds, cashews, flaxseeds, hempseeds, borage oil, primrose oil, cold pressed extra virgin olive oil, grapeseed oil, fish oils, avocado slices, healthy nut butters such as cashew, almond, soy or peanut butter. • 7–10 nuts • 1 tsp. of olive oil • 1/4 avocado • 1 tbsp. of natural nut butter
Any fruit with the exclusion of dates, raisins or candied fruit. Optimal fruit sources are: blueberries raspberries strawberries blackberries cranberries cherries kiwi fruits oranges grapefruits apples bananas peaches pears	Dairy products such as 1% or skim milk, low-fat yogurt with active bacteria, low-fat cheese or cottage cheese. • 1 ounce of cheese	Occasional use of butter • 1 tsp

Continued

Pick 1—Slow Carbohydrates	Pick 2—Lean Proteins	Pick 3—Essential Fats
nectarines apricots pineapples cantaloupes mangoes		
Whole grain food items such as whole rye, barley, oats, quinoa, brown rice, whole wheat and whole grain pasta or bread, kamut, spelt, flax bread, multigrain bread		
Beans—lentils, chickpeas, black beans, etc.		

It is important to note that fats are considerably more dense in calories. When thinking in terms of fat, think of sprinkling this precious macronutrient. Use fat conservatively by sprinkling nuts on a salad, using oil in a salad dressing or adding a spoonful of flaxseed oil to a morning shake.

Examples of Meals or Snacks Using the Pick-3 System

1. **Blueberry banana smoothie**

   Combine ½ banana, ¼ cup of frozen blueberries or mixed berries, ¼ cup of Greek yogurt or 1 scoop of protein powder, ½ cup of almond milk and 1 tbsp. of flaxseed oil. Blend on high.

   Protein—Greek yogurt or protein powder
   Carbohydrate—Blueberries, banana
   Fat—Flaxseed oil

2. **Egg white omelet with broccoli and low-fat cheese** Cook with 1 tsp of butter, 4 pasteurized egg whites, 1 egg, ¼ cup of broccoli florets and 2 ounces of low-fat cheese. Add butter to frying pan and cook over medium heat. Enjoy with a piece of whole grain bread!

Protein–Egg whites, egg, low-fat cheese
Carbohydrate–Broccoli, whole grain toast
Fat–Butter and egg

3. **Bagel lox and cream cheese**
Whole grain bagel, 4 ounces of smoked lox (salmon) and low-fat or dairy-free cream cheese—2 tbsp. Enjoy with ½ handful of almonds.

Protein–Smoked salmon and low-fat cheese
Carbohydrate–Whole grain bagel
Fat–Almonds, some fat in low-fat cheese and in salmon

4. **Slow-cooking oats with mixed berries and walnuts** Add soy milk and/or protein powder—⅓ cup of slow cooking oats, ¾ cup of water, ¼ cup of soy milk, 1 scoop of protein powder, ½ cup of mixed berries, ½ handful of crushed walnuts.

Pour water into saucepan and place on high to boil. Add slow-cooking oats and stir. Bring mixture to a boil again, then reduce heat and simmer for 10–15 minutes. Remove from heat. Add mixed berries and soy milk to cooked oatmeal. Add in protein powder and mix thoroughly. Sprinkle walnuts on top.

Protein–Soy milk or protein powder
Carbohydrate–Oats, berries
Fat–Walnuts

5. Tuna sandwich on multigrain bread with avocado slices

2 slices of whole grain bread, 4 ounces of canned light tuna, ¼ avocado sliced. Add mustard, olive oil, yogurt or small amount of mayonnaise to tuna if desired.

Protein–Tuna
Carbohydrate–Whole grain bread
Fat–Avocado

6. Egg wrap

(Note: eggs have enough fat on their own–fat does not have to be added to whole eggs. I recommend mixing omega-3 eggs and egg whites when using eggs.) ½ whole egg, 2 egg whites, 1 whole grain wrap, ¼ shredded romaine lettuce, ⅛ cup diced tomatoes, salt, pepper, 1 tbsp. mild salsa.

Mix egg and egg whites. Cook in non-stick pan until fully cooked. Toast wrap over burner or under broiler in oven. Place cooked egg in center of wrap, top with lettuce, tomato and salsa. Wrap and serve.

Protein–Egg white
Carbohydrate–Whole grain wrap, tomato, salsa
Fat–Egg yolk

7. Walnut-crusted salmon with broccoli and sweet potatoes

5 ounces of wild Atlantic salmon fillet, skin removed, 1 cup broccoli florets, 1 medium sweet potato, peeled, 1 tbsp. crushed walnuts, 1 tsp. olive oil, ½ tsp. dillseed, ¼ fresh lemon, 2 tbsp. light soy sauce, salt and pepper.

Brush salmon with olive oil, and sprinkle on dillseed, salt, pepper and juice from ¼ fresh lemon. Place in non-stick pan and broil for 8 minutes.

Peel and slice sweet potato and place in non-stick frying pan with broccoli with a small amount of water. Cover and cook for 10 minutes on medium high. Uncover, add soy sauce and cook for another 2 minutes. Serve on plate with salmon.

Protein–Salmon
Carbohydrate–Sweet potato and broccoli
Fat–Olive oil

8. Spelt pasta with tomato sauce, olive oil and chicken breast

¾ cup spelt pasta, ¼ cup of your favorite tomato sauce, 1 tbsp. olive oil, ¼ white onion—diced, 1 whole skinless, boneless chicken breast, 1 tsp. poultry seasoning, salt and pepper.

Bring 1 liter of water to a boil in a pot, add in spelt pasta and cook al dente (approx. 8 minutes). Cut chicken breast coated in poultry seasoning into small strips. Drain pasta, place olive oil in non-stick frying pan, add onions and diced chicken and sauté until chicken is fully cooked. Add pasta and sauce to mixture. Simmer for 10 minutes and serve.

Protein–Chicken
Carbohydrate–Spelt pasta, tomato sauce
Fat–Olive oil

As you can see, in certain recipes such as the blueberry banana smoothie, I have used a combination of slow carbohydrates (½ banana and ¼ cup of berries) and a mixture of proteins (¼ cup of Greek yogurt and ½ cup of almond milk). This is totally acceptable and will achieve the same results. As long as you have one selection of each macronutrient—proteins, fats and carbohydrates per meal and/or snack—you will maintain proper blood sugar control. This, in turn, will enable you to feel energetic and will enable you to lose any excess weight.

To demonstrate the flexibility and variety that this system offers, refer to the recipe section at the back of the book.

THE AMOUNT OF GRAIN TO EAT ON THE PICK-3 SYSTEM

I have been fortunate enough to have enormous clinical experience with weight loss. In my three clinics, my nutritionists and I have had the pleasure of working with thousands of clients to help them lose weight successfully (and I myself lost 75 pounds after having my first child!). Because of this experience, what works and what does not work becomes abundantly clear. What I know for sure is that there are certain nutritional habits that are an absolute must when it comes to losing weight. They are not hard in any way; they just take some getting used to. And once you do "click into" these habits, you have the luxury of indulging more in other areas.

In short, two very basic nutritional practices to follow for quick and sustained weight loss results are:

1. Most days, do not eat your grain after your afternoon snack (i.e., 3 to 4 p.m.).
2. Make dinner your lightest meal.

Consider the following study. Recently, researchers in Tel Aviv demonstrated that eating a higher-calorie breakfast and a lower-calorie dinner helped with weight loss and also reduced the risk of developing diabetes and high blood pressure. The subjects (93 in total) were split into two groups, both consuming a 1400-calorie diet of the same proteins, fats and carbohydrates.

The key difference was that the first group ate a 700-calorie breakfast, a 500-calorie lunch and a 200-calorie dinner. The second group ate the most calories at dinner (i.e., they reversed their caloric intake). The results demonstrate that weight loss is not just about mathematics or calories (finally... I have been saying this for years!). In a three-month period, the first group lost 17.8 pounds on average while the second group lost only 7.3 pounds. In addition, the first group did not want to snack later in the day and had no blood sugar (glucose) spikes. Take-home point ... front-load your day with food! You do not have to go as light as eating a 200-calorie dinner, but dinner should not be your heaviest meal. As the old saying goes, "Eat breakfast like a king, lunch like a prince and dinner like a pauper."

While this study helps to solidify one of the ways I have been practicing weight loss for years, I also realize that the task of eating in a lighter fashion after 3 p.m. is easier said than done. Oftentimes, we overeat at dinner (or after dinner) due to stress, fatigue, lack of time or intense sugar cravings. In order to get into the habit of eating lighter as the day goes on, I recommend:

- Eliminating your grain in the evening. Aim to have your grain at breakfast (i.e., cereal), lunch (i.e., a sandwich on sprouted-grain bread) or afternoon snack.

- Eat a sufficient amount of protein at dinner so you are not hungry. For women, this is a minimum of 3 to 5 ounces of protein per meal; for men, it is 4 to 6 ounces of protein. For eyeballing purposes, 3 ounces of protein is about the size of the palm of your hand (without your fingers or thumb).

- Keep free foods around to grab. All of your vegetables, such as baby carrots, peppers, broccoli, cucumbers, radishes, Brussels sprouts, tomatoes, and cauliflower, are free. You can eat as much as you like whenever you like. Please note: Potatoes, squash and corn are not considered "free vegetables."

- If hungry, opt for a little bit more of the "good fat" foods such as almonds, walnuts, avocados, and olive oil. The good fat will fill you up without affecting your weight loss results.

- Drink your water. Oftentimes we mistake hunger and thirst for each other. Make sure you are well hydrated throughout your day and after dinner (2.5 liters per day).

- Opt for two Dr. Joey's Skinnychews. With 2 grams of prebiotic inulin fiber per chew, they are the perfect dark-chocolaty option for after-dinner cravings or hunger. For more information, please visit www.drjoey.com.

Once you understand how to use the Pick-3 System of eating, the mystery of losing weight, keeping it off and feeling great will finally be revealed. You will be empowered to control your weight on your own for the rest of your life, and you will never need another diet book or program again.

The steps outlined in this chapter will provide the flexibility to eat the foods you love, all the while obtaining your health goals. Remember, if you fall off the health wagon and indulge from time to time, that's okay—I even encourage it! The key is to follow the principles outlined in the nourish step most of the time (80 percent) and save the "no-no" foods for weekends, holidays and celebrations.

Summary of Step 2 — Nourish

1. Forget low carb—eat slow carb!
2. Consume lean proteins at every meal or snack.
3. Eat essential fats.
4. Follow the Pick-3 System of eating (it keeps your metabolism revved!).

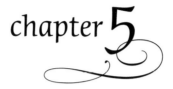

chapter 5

STEP 3—MOISTURIZE

"Health is so necessary to all the duties, as well as the pleasure of life, that the crime of squandering it is equal to the folly."

—SAMUEL JOHNSON

The body thrives both internally and externally when it is in an environment that promotes moisture. Put simply, there are several external factors that rob moisture from the body: seasonal changes, lack of water in the diet, lack of plant nutrients, smoking and continual use of diuretics such as coffee and alcohol. Although these factors are significant in decreasing the amount of moisture in your body, none is more critical than the deficiency of omega-3 fats in the diet. Similar to the way a conditioner works on a hair follicle, omega-3 fats maintain proper elasticity and moisture to all organs in the body including the digestive system, skin and hair. Signs and symptoms of omega-3 deficiency include dry hair and skin (i.e., a "goosebump" rash on skin), brittle nails, excessive thirst, frequent urination, fatigue, attention problems and an inability to lose weight.

Omega-3 fats have been gaining more and more press recently due to the tremendous health benefits that have been substantiated by literally hundreds of research studies. Of the numerous roles they play in the body, these precious fats have been shown to help protect against and in some cases even reverse the ill effects of the following health conditions:

- Heart disease
- High cholesterol
- High blood pressure
- Acne
- Arthritis
- Asthma
- Attention deficit disorder
- Breast cancer
- Inflammatory bowel disease (Crohn's disease and ulcerative colitis)

- Raynaud's syndrome and lupus
- Depression
- Menstrual pains
- Multiple sclerosis
- Epilepsy
- Neurological conditions
- Fibromyalgia
- Chronic fatigue syndrome
- Weight management

> **Food Fact:** It is estimated that 85 percent or more people in the Western world are deficient in omega-3 fatty acids, while most get far too much of the omega-6 fatty acids.

Omega-3 Food Options

Alpha-linolenic acid (ALA) as well as the fatty acids *eicosapentaenoic acid* (EPA) and *docosahexaenoic acid* (DHA) all belong to a group of fatty acids called omega-3 fatty acids. The omega-3 fats are called essential fats because they cannot be made by the body, and therefore they must be acquired from the food you eat. EPA and DHA are found primarily in cold-water fish sources, while ALA is highly concentrated in certain plant oils such as flaxseed oil and to a lesser extent in canola, soy and walnut oils. Once ingested, the body converts ALA to EPA and DHA, the two types of omega-3 fatty acids more readily used by the body.

> **Food Fact:** Walnuts, which are rich in omega-3 fat, have been shown to lower cholesterol and triglycerides in people with high cholesterol.

Due to the ingestion of too many omega-6 fats in the form of refined vegetable oils, a majority of North Americans are critically deficient in omega-3 fats. While our ancestors ate a diet that contained a ratio of omega-6 to omega-3 of about 1:1, due to food processing and manufacturing, the current ratio is something closer to about 20:1. It is this skewed ratio of omega-6 to omega-3 fats that is mainly responsible for the inflammatory effects that occur in the body. Too many of the wrong inflammatory fats and too few omega-3 fats are both root causes in numerous chronic diseases that are prevalent today, including arthritis, heart disease, cancer, asthma, skin conditions, obesity and depression. Remember, chronic and long-lasting inflammation is one of the three beauty robbers that prematurely steal your inner health and outer beauty (see chapter 2). To ward off unnecessary inflammatory effects and to have your skin and body look its best begin by reducing the amount of processed vegetable oils in the diet and supplementing with the proper sources of omega-3 foods and supplements. When using omega-6 fats, eliminate or minimize the vegetable oils such as sunflower, safflower and sesame oil and select higher-quality sources of omega-6 fats such as borage oil, black current oil or primrose oil. Although borage, black current and primrose oils are classified as omega-6, these oils are rich in gamma linolenic acid (GLA) and do not have the same inflammatory effects that safflower, sunflower and sesame oil do. In fact, the GLA found in borage, black current and primrose oil has anti-inflammatory effects that have been shown to be beneficial for promoting heart health, improving skin conditions and lowering cholesterol. Refer to table 5.1 on common sources of fats and table 5.2 for food sources of omega-3.

Food Fact: The average Canadian only ingests 130 mg of combined EPA/DHA per day. Adults should ingest between 2–3 grams of EPA/DHA daily.

Table 5.1: Common Sources of Fat

Family Name	Common Name	Food Source
Omega-9	Oleic acid	Canola, olive, and peanut oils, animal products, avocado
Omega-6	Linoleic acid	Corn, safflower, soybean, cottonseed, and sunflower oils (the pro-inflammatory oils) Borage, black current and primrose oils (the anti-inflammatory oils that contain GLA)
	Arachadonic acid	Animal products
Omega-3	Alpha-linolenic acid	Canola and soybean oils, some nuts, flaxseed
	Eicosapentaenoic acid	Fish and fish oils
	Docosahexainoic acid	Fish and fish oils

Food Fact: Low levels of omega-3 fatty acids are associated with depression and other psychological/neurological conditions.

Table 5.2: Food Sources of Omega-3

Food Source	Milligrams of Omega-3
1 teaspoon of flaxseed oil	2500 mg
1/4 cup of walnuts	2000 mg
4 ounces of Atlantic salmon	2800 mg
4 ounces of tuna	2600 mg
4 ounces of mackerel	1800 mg
Omega-3 egg	300–400 mg

What about Flaxseeds?

Flaxseeds and flaxseed oil offer a wonderful source of omega-3. One option is to use flaxseed oil in salad dressings or to sprinkle ground flaxseeds into a morning shake or juice, or on cereal or a salad. Yet, in terms of reaping the proper amount of EPA and DHA from flaxseed, the results show that flaxseed is just not enough. Although the major type of fat present in flaxseed oil, ALA, can be converted to EPA and DHA (the two types of omega-3 fat more readily absorbed by the body), for the majority of people, the conversion appears to be inefficient. For example, fish oil has been shown to have anti-inflammatory effects for conditions such as rheumatoid arthritis, while the effects of flaxseed oil on inflammation are inconclusive. Fish oil has also been shown to reduce platelet aggregation (the stickiness of your blood cells), which is a risk factor for heart disease; however, flaxseed oil did not demonstrate the same results. There are some health benefits that have been associated with the use of ground flaxseeds or flaxseed oil, such as reduced cholesterol and help with constipation.

In summary, flaxseed oil or ground flaxseeds are a wonderful addition to any diet and should be used daily. However, they should not be relied on as a source of omega-3 due to their inefficient conversion to EPA and DHA. When using flaxseed oil, never heat it. It is not suitable for cooking and should always be stored in an opaque, airtight container in the refrigerator or freezer. If the oil has a noticeable odor, it is probably rancid and should be discarded.

Whole flaxseeds can be purchased at most bulk food or health food stores. The outer husks are very hard and difficult to crack when chewing. Because of this, whole flaxseeds must be ground up in a coffee grinder, food processor or blender so you can digest them. If not, whole flaxseeds will pass right through the body undigested, losing all of their nutritional advantage. By grinding them, you will benefit from the fiber, essential oils and *lignans* (beneficial plant chemicals) present. Similar to grinding coffee, I recommend grinding your flaxseeds quite fine for the best palatability. To ensure freshness, after grinding, store your flaxseeds in an airtight, dark container. Ground flaxseeds stay fresh and safe to eat for 90 days.

Food Fact: Research suggests you need to take almost 10 times the amount of flaxseed oil to get the equivalent amount of DHA and EPA found in fish oils. Approximately 7.2 grams of flaxseed oil is equivalent to the benefits of 1 gram of fish oil.

FLAXSEED OIL SALAD DRESSING

- 2 tablespoons extra virgin olive oil
- 1 tablespoon flaxseed oil
- 1 tablespoon white balsamic vinegar
- 1 teaspoon lemon juice
- 2 tablespoons capers
- ½ teaspoon fresh chopped garlic
- Salt and freshly ground black pepper to taste

In a small bowl, whisk together the olive oil, flaxseed oil, vinegar, lemon juice, chopped garlic and capers. Season with salt and pepper.

The Safety of Fish

There are pros and cons when it comes to eating fish these days. The pros are that fish are a wonderful source of protein and are low in saturated fat, and the cold-water type offer a good source of omega-3 fatty acids. The cons of eating fish have to do with their toxicity level. With tuna, one of the most highly eaten fish, the concern lies with the amount of mercury present in the fish. It is estimated that mercury levels in the environment have increased three to five times in the past century due to industrial operations such as pulp and paper processing, burning garbage and fossil fuels, mining operations and releases from dental offices. Mercury is toxic in all its forms. In fish, mercury appears in the form of methyl mercury, which can be very damaging to the nervous system. Effects can range from learning disorders and developmental delays to headaches, migraines, muscle aches, depression, memory loss, skin rashes and seizures. Mercury accumulation is a grave concern for pregnant or nursing mothers due to the dangerous neurological effects mercury can have on a fetus or infant. Large predator fish, such as swordfish, king mackerel, tilefish and shark, which feed on smaller fish, all have a greater chance of accumulating methyl mercury because of their longer lifespan. If you experience any of the above symptoms without a cause and suspect you may have higher than acceptable amounts of mercury in your system, have your doctor conduct a heavy metal test of your blood, urine or hair. If you test positive, follow a heavy metal detoxification plan under the supervision of a qualified healthcare practitioner.

In March 2004, the Food and Drug Administration (FDA) and the Environmental Protection Agency (EPA) announced their revised consumer advisory on fish and mercury consumption. Here are their recommendations for pregnant women, nursing mothers and young children:

1. Do not eat shark, swordfish, king mackerel, or tilefish because they contain high levels of mercury.

2. Eat up to 12 ounces (2 average portions) a week of a variety of fish and shellfish that are lower in mercury.

   - The five most commonly eaten fish that are low in mercury are shrimp, canned light tuna, salmon, pollock and catfish.
   - Another commonly eaten fish, albacore ("white") tuna has more mercury than canned light tuna. So, when choosing your two meals of fish and shellfish, you may eat up to 6 ounces (one average meal) of albacore tuna per week.

3. Check local advisories about the safety of fish caught in your local lakes, rivers, and coastal areas. If no advice is available, eat up to 6 ounces (one average portion) per week of fish you catch from local waters, but don't consume any other fish during that week.

Due to the changing nature of fish recommendations and the ever-continuing rising levels of mercury, I am more conservative than the EPA and FDA in the amounts of fish I eat and recommend to my family, friends and patients.

> **Food Fact:** Tuna is a favorite fish, appearing in over 90 percent of households. In fact, approximately 20 percent of U.S. fish consumption is of tuna. Children and pregnant women eat more than twice as much tuna as any other fish.

WHAT ABOUT TUNA?

According to a study conducted by a public interest group, the Mercury Policy Project, mercury levels were 30 percent higher than the tuna industry had previously reported. Of the 48 tunas sampled, over three were found to contain mercury levels considerably higher than the Food and Drug Administration's recommendations. They concluded from their results that one of every 20 cans of white or albacore tuna should be recalled as being unsafe for human consumption. Because we don't know the actual amount of mercury we are consuming when we eat tuna, I recommend pregnant women and nursing mothers consume no more than 6 ounces of light tuna per month. For everyone else, 6 ounces of canned light (not white) tuna per week appears to be safe.

Food Fact: About 6 percent of women of childbearing age have levels of mercury above those deemed safe by the Environmental Protection Agency.

WHAT ABOUT SALMON?

In an attempt to avoid the mercury found in tuna, many fish lovers have turned to salmon as a healthy option. The upside is that salmon is full of protein and omega-3 heart-healthy fats. The downside is that farmed salmon is not as healthy as we once thought. According to several recent studies, farmed salmon contains unsafe levels of dioxins and PCBs. Dioxins and PCBs are chemicals formed by unwanted by-products in a variety of industrial processes. They are found throughout the environment, and fish accumulate them primarily by eating other fish or fish feed. PCBs have not been used since the 1970s, but they continue to persist in the environment. Dioxins and PCBs have been linked to several serious health conditions such as liver damage, immune system suppression and developmental delay in children.

In a large-scale study reported in 2004, the average dioxin level in farm-raised salmon was 11 times higher than in wild salmon. The study also reported the average PCB levels were 36.6 parts per billion (ppb) in farm-raised salmon, versus 4.75 ppb in wild salmon. In response to this study, the World Health Organization (WHO) released the following statement:

> *WHO consider[s] fish to be an important component of a nutritious diet, and that the risk of consuming contaminated fish must be weighted in view of the beneficial nutritive effects of fish. FAO [Food and Agriculture Organization of the United Nations] and WHO plan to develop general guidance for such risk-benefit considerations, with the contamination of fish as case studies.*

In my analysis of the situation, this statement is ridiculous and irresponsible. We should not have to weigh the risk-benefit ratio of eating particular foods. Instead, we should eat the cleanest and safest foods possible. We should also design new methods for farmers to clean up their fish farming so that they produce healthy, risk-free fish. Healthy environments and safer feed for farmed salmon are easy to initiate; such new approaches should be required and implemented by responsible farmers immediately. If done correctly, this transition would not cost fish farmers more. In fact, they would likely reap more business and profits from the positive consumer attention that providing a safer product would attract. We do not have the luxury of time to study the ill effects that dioxins and PCBs will have on your family or mine—the time for change is now.

> A study reported in 2004 in the journal *Chemosphere* found the level of PCBs in farmed salmon in the United States and Canada to be five to 10 times higher than those in wild salmon.

When it comes to diet, you have the greatest influence on your health and the health of your family. Gather the facts from food organizations and agencies, critically assess them and then make a decision that feels right for you. In the case of salmon, instead of following the ludicrous recommendation of weighing risk-benefit considerations of food, it is best to purchase "cleaner" wild or organic salmon. I realize this option is more expensive, but with enough consumer demand and pressure, the price will soon fall. In addition to having a significantly lower toxic load, wild salmon tastes better. Once you eat a fillet or smoked wild Atlantic salmon (lox), you will instantly notice the difference in color, taste and texture.

> **Food Fact:** Scientists have observed that countries with the highest rates of depression, post-partum depression, and seasonal affective disorder (SAD) have lower intakes of dietary fish.

FISH OIL SUPPLEMENTS

As with eating fish, the safety of consuming fish oils has also come under the microscope. With the fish pollutant scares, many have become concerned that fish oils may also contain dangerous PCBs and dioxins. The good news is this: for the most part, they do not. You can now gain all the benefits of eating fish without the toxicity by supplementing with fish oils.

ConsumerLab.com, a company designed to independently test various supplements, vitamins and other health products, tested 41 various types of fish oil capsules for the presence of toxins. Of all the capsules tested, none contained detectable levels of PCBs or dioxins. In another study, conducted by the *Globe and Mail* (a Canadian national newspaper) in conjunction with CTV (a Canadian network), it was found that:

> A person would need to consume as many as 312 fish oil capsules to be exposed to the amount of polychlorinated biphenyls in a single serving of farmed salmon. Even the cleanest serving of farmed fish had as much PCB as 63 fish oil capsules. A serving of wild salmon, which is much less contaminated than farmed fish, had the same PCB content as about 20 capsules.

PICKING A FISH OIL SUPPLEMENT

Due to the concerns with fish and toxicity, I highly recommend continuing to supplement with a minimum of 2–3 grams of fish oils per day to ensure you are getting a sufficient amount of clean omega-3 fats. Including a high-quality source of fish oils in your daily supplement regime is the best way to reap the internal and external benefits that are offered by omega-3 fats without exposure to toxic elements. In a very short time (typically 2 weeks), you will notice the external benefits of taking fish oil supplements: flawless, healthy-looking skin and shiny hair. You will also likely notice an improvement in your digestive capacity. When purchasing a fish oil, you want to ensure the product has three main components:

1. It has been molecularly distilled to ensure its purity.
2. It is derived from smaller fish. Remember: the smaller the fish, the shorter the lifespan and, therefore, the less accumulation of toxins.
3. It is enteric coated to ward off any "fishy repeat" and optimizes digestion of the oil.

FISH OILS AND WEIGHT LOSS

I have heard from many people who are concerned about taking fish oil supplements; they fear they will gain weight from the excess calories found in fats. Do not be concerned about gaining weight from supplementing with these types of fats. Research has shown that omega-3 fats help promote weight loss and are necessary for the body to shift towards a leaner, healthier you. In fact, when dieting, you lose omega-3 fats from your body stores before any other type of fat. Omega-3s are also most readily available and utilized as an energy source versus other types of fats such as saturated fats. Saturated fats are typically stored in the body and are much more difficult to shed. In fact, omega-3s and the good source of omega-6 fat GLA promote weight loss by:

- Increasing *thermogenesis*—the generation or production of heat that promotes weight loss
- Decreasing body fat mass and fat cell volume
- Reducing the amount of calories consumed
- Increasing the storage of fat into lean muscle areas versus saturated fat which is preferentially stored in the abdomen

- Increasing the ability to maintain weight loss
- Turning on genes that may be associated with the inhibition of abdominal obesity
- Regulating the activity of the area of the brain responsible for the perception of fullness (satiety)

Summary of Step 3 — Moisturize

- Include omega-3 foods such as walnuts, flaxseed oil and a moderate amount of high-quality fish in your daily diet.
- Avoid omega-6 pro-inflammatory oils such as safflower, sunflower and sesame oils.
- Include the anti-inflammatory omega-6 oils such as borage, black current and primrose oil.
- Consume 2–3 grams of high-quality fish oil supplements daily.

chapter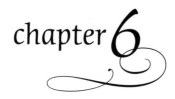

STEP 4—MAINTENANCE

"A wise man should consider that health is the greatest of human blessings."

—HIPPOCRATES

*B*y this point, you have successfully completed your five-day cleanse, are eating according to the Pick-3 System of eating and are supplementing daily with 2–3 grams of high-quality fish oils. The food behaviors recommended in this chapter have nothing to do with "what" you eat, rather it deals with "how" you eat. This chapter offers new approaches to eating that will allow you to eat as much as you like during the day without encountering weight gain or setbacks in health. By following the four elements outlined below, you will be able to maintain the health changes you have already witnessed and propel yourself even further into the optimal "health groove." After a short time, these practices will become habit and you will notice additional health advances such as a significant improvement in digestion, a naturally flatter stomach, an even greater burst in your daily energy and best of all—the ability to stop counting calories!

The four elements involved in the maintenance step are:

1. Do not eat past 7 p.m., with the exception of free food.
2. Eat until you are sufficiently full—not stuffed!
3. Eat three meals and one snack daily.
4. Do not count calories.

Element #1 — Do Not Eat Past 7 p.m., with the Exception of Free Foods

Not eating past 7 p.m. sounds quite easy, doesn't it? For most people, this change is the hardest step of my plan. Because of the way most people live and work, eating past 7 p.m. is often a reality. After putting the kids to sleep or rushing home from work, it is not uncommon for people to mindlessly munch their dinner at 8, 9 or 10 o'clock at night! After-dinner eating or drinking as a "reward" or for stress relief is also extremely common. Unfortunately, this is a one-way ticket to weight gain and faulty digestion. As mentioned, not only does your metabolism slow as the lights go down, eating late at night can also create a number of health problems. If you refer to the three beauty robbers discussed in chapter 2, you will remember that faulty digestion can be the underlying cause of several symptoms such as a poor complexion, dry skin, hair that lacks luster or is falling out, and bags under the eyes. By changing your habit of late-night munching and not eating from 7 p.m. to 7 a.m. (with the exception of free foods), you are allowing yourself to have a daily "mini-cleanse." By doing so, you allow your digestive juices to burn up any waste that your body needs to get rid of. Whenever considering total health, whether it is inner wellness or outer beauty and radiance, cleaning out the pipes, i.e., the digestive system, is a key component.

When I first began the practice of not eating past dinnertime, I have to be honest—I found it quite difficult. Like many people, I was an emotional eater who turned to food after my kids were asleep as a sweet reward at the end of my day. However, in order to reap the benefits of eating only free foods after dinner, there are a few simple steps that can help. They are:

1. Turn to your free foods to mindlessly munch. Your free foods include all vegetables with the exception of potatoes (white and sweet), peas, corn and squash. In other words, feel free to munch on the following vegetables (in limitless quantities): carrots, broccoli, peppers, cauliflower, cucumbers, radishes, celery, lettuce and cherry tomatoes. I find red peppers and cherry tomatoes especially helpful when having a sweet

craving. These low-calorie, nutrient-dense foods will not hinder your digestive capacity or ability to lose weight in any way.

2. Keep your cupboard well stocked with a variety of herbal teas (lemon, blueberry, peach, strawberry, etc.). When you feel the urge to eat, have a cup of tea instead.

3. Try drinking a glass of water. Oftentimes we mistake our hunger and thirst signals.

4. Fill up on two Skinnychews, which provide a long "mouth feel." To make them last even longer, keep them in the freezer.

5. If you know you will be working late, pack a healthy meal for dinner or plan ahead.

6. Think 80–20. Even if you stop eating by 7 p.m. five times per week, your body will thank you.

Late-night eating often goes hand in hand with emotions and feelings—happy, bored, sad, lonely—we eat! Our relationship with food is often one of the most powerful relationships we develop early in life. It is also one of the hardest to change because unlike alcohol, drugs or cigarettes, food cannot be eliminated completely, of course. We simply have to make the shift to create a peaceful relationship with our food choices.

When first starting to change a food behavior, it takes focus, mindfulness, willpower and a look into the "why" of your eating patterns. In other words, what are your triggers? Are they situational or rooted deeper than that? Luckily, physical and mental health are intertwined. Thus, when you start to make nutritional changes and eat better, you will soon start to feel better about your appearance and your body. Throw some cardiovascular activity and weight training into that equation and voila … things start to slowly shift. I encourage all of my clients to follow the plan outlined in this book for at least 30 days (keeping a food journal, making better choices, reducing grain and after-dinner eating, etc.). My entire goal is to get you "addicted" to feeling better. If you fall off the health wagon and eat or even binge in the first 30 days, do not panic. This is common and happens. Simply dust off your knees, put your chin up and continue on. I assure you … you can do it. You can make the shift.

Additional strategies to dealing with your engrained patterns of emotional eating include:

1. Institute a replacement behavior for your eating. You cannot eliminate one behavior in the long term without substituting something else in its place. Whether it is working out, drinking water or herbal tea, chewing gum, brushing your teeth or recording your thoughts in a journal—just keep at it!

2. Identify your cues. There are certain triggers that typically cause you to overeat to soothe emotions. Perhaps speaking to your mother-in-law on the phone or arguing with your boyfriend trigger you. Whatever the reason, identify the cue and then substitute eating with your replacement behavior.

3. Do not, I repeat—*do not*—keep unhealthy munchies in your kitchen cupboards or fridge. When an emotional situation arises that challenges you (and I assure you, it always does), those chocolate chip cookies or ice cream will be far too tempting. Part of the steps to healing inside and out is undergoing a "kitchen audit." Put this book down and go to your cupboards and fridge and remove all refined carbohydrates and snack foods such as cookies, cereal, candy, ice cream, pretzels, chips, nachos and other goodies from your cupboards. Start stocking your kitchen with healthier snacks for

you and your family: raw nuts, seeds, fruits, vegetables, yogurt and whole grain foods. If you feel yourself sliding into a food binge, grab sliced cucumbers or mini carrots. The action of chewing and swallowing should help you get over the urge to eat.

4. Open up. Whether it is to a friend or a qualified therapist, talk to someone you trust about what is bothering you. In addition to journaling or meditating, you must have an outlet for what is troubling you.

Element #2 — Eat Until You Are Sufficiently Full — Not Stuffed!

"Never eat more than you can lift."

—Miss Piggy

In North America, we are experiencing what I refer to as "portion distortion." In other words, we are consuming more calories than we ever have. No longer are deficiency syndromes such as rickets (a lack of vitamin D) or scurvy (a lack of vitamin C) a reality. In contrast, our major disease epidemics of the twenty-first century are "gluttony diseases" such as heart disease, obesity, cancer and stroke. Common selling slogans such as "two for one," "all you can eat" and "supersized" are all lures that are causing consumers to eat more and more without even realizing it. To top it off, a majority of processed and fast foods are laced with flavor enhancers such as MSG (monosodium glutamate) that trigger our brains to increase our appetite. Consequently, a majority of people today have become completely out of tune with their true hunger signals and eat to the point of being completely stuffed, bloated and uncomfortable. Common symptoms that we are eating too much and clogging the pipes of our digestive system include acid reflux, constipation, burping, bloating and heartburn.

In addition to our digestive systems taking a hit, recent studies have shown that eating too many of the wrong foods such as refined carbohydrates, saturated fats and trans fatty acids are also precursors to the other two beauty robbers: 1) inflammation and 2) free radical damage. In a study published in 2004, subjects were given a 930-calorie meal that consisted of a McDonald's Egg McMuffin, a Sausage McMuffin and two hash browns. Eating this highly processed food showed extreme negative effects on the participants' arteries and therefore their blood flow. This effect lasted for longer than 3 hours following the meal.

According to the study's co-author, Dr. Paresh Dandona, chief of endocrinology at State University of New York:

> ... *certain types of nutrients, most notably fats and carbohydrate sugars, appeared to induce the release of free radical damage (cellular damage), which in turn triggered inflammation. Compared to individuals who had received no breakfast, those who had eaten the McDonald's meal displayed evidence of free radical generation by the circulating white blood cells, which would cause inflammation within the white blood cells.*

Here are three steps to follow to become more aware of how much you are eating and to once again get in tune with your hunger signals:

1. **Let yourself get hungry.** Do not eat according to the clock. Prior to eating a meal or snack, be sure you actually feel that "grumbling in your stomach." I promise you, you will not starve. Rather, you will become in tune with your body's true sensation of hunger.

2. **Slow down and focus.** It takes a minimum of 20 minutes for the stretch receptors in the stomach to register a "full sensation" in the brain. In other words, if you shovel in a lot of food in under 10 minutes—the average time of the North American meal—you will tend to overeat. I recommend practicing "mindful eating." In other words, slow down your meals by sitting at a table, using utensils to eat and taking sips of water or breathing between bites. Although on occasion there is no avoiding it, eating in front of the television or computer or in your car is not a good habit to get into.

3. **Eat foods filled with protein.** Foods that are filled with fiber, protein and good fat are more filling and will give you that full sensation earlier on in comparison to other foods. Fiber-filled foods include raw fruits, vegetables, whole grains, ground flaxseeds, bran and beans, while the "good" fat foods include olive oil, avocados and high-quality nuts such as walnuts, almonds or cashews. Protein options include chicken, turkey, eggs, red meat, protein powder (rice, hemp, pea or soy), Greek yogurt and cottage cheese.

Food Fact: Thanks to supersized portions, the total calorie content of a typical fast food meal of cheeseburger, fries and Coke has been hoisted to 1340 calories from 680 calories. That is more than half a normal recommended daily calorie consumption.

Once you slow down, practice mindful eating and eat healthy fiber-, fat- or protein-filled foods, you will find you eat until you are sufficiently full, not stuffed! Benjamin Franklin had the best advice when he said, "To lengthen thy life, lessen thy meals."

It is also a good idea to become familiar with the average serving sizes of foods. Refer to table 6.1 for general guidelines.

A supersized soft drink (42 ounces) contains 136 grams of sugar which is equivalent to 34 teaspoons of sugar!

Table 6.1 Nutritional Content of Sample Serving Sizes

Carbohydrates	Proteins	Fats
• 1 serving of fruit (1/2 cup or 1 small fruit) = 10 grams	• 4 ounces of chicken or fish = 28 grams	• 1/8 of an avocado = 5 grams
• 1 cup of vegetables = 5 grams	• 3 ounces of sirloin steak = 25 grams	• 1 tablespoon of peanut butter = 5 grams
• 1/2 cup of beans = 20–25 grams	• 1/2 cup of egg whites = 13 grams	
• 1 whole wheat tortilla = 12 grams	• 1 ounce of low-fat cheese = 7 grams	
• 2 pieces of crisp Wasa bread = 15 grams	• 4 ounces of firm tofu = 10 grams	
• 1 slice of bread (whole wheat) = 15 grams		
• 1 bagel = 25–40 grams of carbohydrates (depending on density)		

Element #3 — Eat Three Meals and One Snack Daily

After several years of analyzing hundreds of personal meal plans submitted to me by my patients, I started to notice a trend. People who were breakfast skippers and late-night eaters were the ones who had the most difficulty losing weight. Even though many of them were doing intensive cardio workouts three to five times per week, not one pound was coming off. To make matters worse, these people (some in their early 20s and 30s!) had poor energy, never woke up feeling rested and had dry, brittle hair, skin and nails as well as digestive complaints.

It is critical to start your day with a balanced meal in order to stabilize your blood sugar levels. The reason breakfast skippers have difficulty losing weight is due to their poor blood sugar control.

Picture this common scenario:

Person A skips breakfast and only has a cup of coffee until one o'clock in the afternoon. The coffee temporarily spikes her glucose (sugar) levels and causes her to oversecrete insulin. Remember, excess insulin triggers the storage of excess fat. By early afternoon, due to low blood sugar and hunger, she is feeling shaky, irritable and fatigued, so she grabs the closest and easiest carbohydrate such as a muffin, pasta, white bread sandwich or chocolate chip cookie to eat. But because her lunch consists of high Glycemic Index carbo-hydrates, her blood sugar levels bounce around; her insulin is once again oversecreted. Once the carbohydrate she has eaten at lunch wears off, her blood sugar levels become too low due to an over-secretion of insulin; she becomes hypoglycemic. Consequently, a craving sets in for more sugary carbohydrates or sweets to get her out of her food fog. After Person A returns home late at night from a busy day at the office, she is famished and fatigued, so she once again grabs the quickest and easiest food or hits the local drive-thru to satisfy her hunger. See how this nasty trend develops? A common combination of breakfast skipping, lack of protein, lack of essential fats and late-night eating is a typical trend that can push you off the path of health.

Now, let's consider a healthier scenario: Person B starts her day with a breakfast from the Pick-3 System of eating. In other words, her breakfast consists of a slow-burning carbohydrate such as whole grain toast, a protein such as an egg or yogurt and good fat such as healthy nut butter. Eating in this manner stabilizes her blood sugar (glucose) control and she secretes a normal amount of insulin. Mood, energy and cravings are all controlled or kept at bay. Person B is also not starving by the time snack time or lunchtime arrives and so she eats sensibly, with control and for hunger reasons—not for cravings or to boost her energy. By eating three meals and one snack, you can maintain your energy and avoid excess weight gain. Your body will receive the proper nourishment for the day—a beautiful scenario!

> If after eating a meal or snack you are tired or "foggy" you have either eaten the wrong food combination (too many carbohydrates), have a sensitivity to a food (for instance, a dairy or wheat allergy) or have eaten too much and have clogged up your digestive system.

The fact that those who skip meals tend to weigh more has been demonstrated by various studies. For example, a recent study published in the *American Journal of Epidemiology* concluded that skipping meals and eating less frequently may result in weight gain. Since more than 60 percent of Americans are overweight and 27 percent are obese, these results are extremely relevant. Consider the following findings:

- Individuals who ate four or more times a day were 45 percent less likely to be obese than those who ate three times a day or less.
- Skipping breakfast was linked with a greater chance of obesity. People who skipped breakfast were more than four times more likely to be obese than those who ate breakfast daily.

So what is the ideal way to eat? For weight loss and optimal health, it is best to eat three meals and one snack daily. I recommend having your snack either between breakfast and lunch, or between lunch and dinner. I find a 4 p.m. snack works best for most people. By eating three meals and one snack and following the Pick-3 System of eating, your blood sugar and insulin response will not undergo a continual roller-coaster ride and you will find yourself feeling satiated, satisfied, free of cravings and energetic.

Element #4 — Do Not Count Calories

I have witnessed far too many patients who severely restrict their caloric intake in an attempt to lose weight and feel great. I have seen a number of people literally starve themselves by going on diets that recommended a mere 600 to 800 caloric intake per day! While this approach may have worked for them temporarily, 99 percent of the time it could not be maintained and resulted in more weight gain, frustration and depression. When calories are extremely restricted, the body, in its innate intelligence, thinks that it is starving and undergoes a mode called the *starvation adaptation mode*. In other words, the body thinks, "I better save up and cling on to all these calories and store them as fat." Not only is severe caloric restriction extremely difficult to maintain and taxing on the system, it is counterproductive because in the long run, you gain more weight.

Although I do not recommend severely restricting your caloric intake, I also do not recommend over consuming calories. A balance can be found between these two choices that does not involve counting calories. While many of us want to know the calorie counts of different types of food, calories have little to do with health. The steps outlined above and in the other chapters are the keys to real success. These patterns of healthy eating and tasty nutritional options pave the way to optimal health and wellness. Instead of counting calories, simply follow the steps outlined in this chapter along with the other strategies in this book to shift your health to its greatest potential.

Summary of Step 4 — Maintenance

- Do not eat past 7 p.m., with the exception of free foods.
- Eat until you are sufficiently full—not stuffed!
- Eat three meals and one snack daily.
- Do not count calories.

Now that you have learned all four steps of the natural makeover diet, the following chapters will offer you health optimizer answers to your commonly asked questions and delicious and easy-to-make recipes. Prior to moving on, let's first review the main points of the 4-step program.

- Step 1—Cleanse for five days (chapter 3).
- Step 2—Nourish by following the Pick-3 System of eating.
- Step 3—Moisturize. Continue to supplement with 2–3 grams of fish oil daily.
- Step 4—Maintain. Get in tune with your body's hunger signals, top load your day with food and do not eat past 7 p.m., with the exception of free foods. Do not count calories and eat three meals and one snack daily.

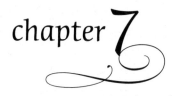

chapter 7

HEALTH OPTIMIZERS

"The road to better health will not be found through more drugs, doctors and hospitals. Instead, it will be discovered through better nutrition and changes in lifestyle."

—WILLIAM CROOK, M.D.

In addition to the four steps outlined in the previous chapters (cleanse, nourish, moisturize and maintenance), there are three health approaches that, when followed, result in powerful health, beauty, energy and weight loss results. The three additional health optimizers are:

1.   Make sleep a priority. Get a minimum of seven hours of quality sleep per day.
2.   Engage in compressive and expansive exercises five days per week.
3.   Get happy!

Health Optimizer #1 — Get a Minimum of Seven Hours of Quality Sleep Per Day

Sleep is the body's most effective method of shutting down to allow recuperation and restorative functions to occur. A good night's sleep keeps the immune system strong and better able to fight off bacteria and viruses, allows the body to better deal with stressors, sharpens mental capacity, lowers the risk of diabetes and heart disease and can even help with weight loss! Yet, at one time or another, due to life stressors, illness or grief we have all experienced a degree of sleep deprivation where we have felt on edge, anxiety stricken, foggy and/or had cravings for sweet, sugary foods. External factors such as light, noise pollution, poor food choices, smoking and alcohol can all cause interrupted sleep. Yet, even if you do manage to sleep through the night, as you will discover, there is more to sleep than merely lying down for six to nine hours. The quality and quantity of sleep you get nightly has a huge impact on how you function and interact during the day and your state of health. How do you know if you are experiencing a mild state of sleep deprivation? Ask yourself the following questions:

1. Do you wake feeling rested?
2. Do you have difficulty falling asleep (longer than 20 minutes)?
3. Do you fall asleep as soon as your head hits the pillow (less than five minutes)?
4. Do you wake up frequently during the night (more than once)?
5. Do you feel tired, depressed and burned-out during your day?
6. Do you have difficulty losing weight?
7. Do you crave sugary foods and/or starchy carbohydrates?

> If it takes you less than five minutes to fall asleep at night, it means you're sleep deprived. The ideal time is between 10 and 15 minutes, which indicates you're still tired enough to sleep deeply, but not so exhausted that you feel sleepy all the time.

It is important to remember that a mild state of sleep deprivation typically goes hand in hand with a highly demanding job, a fast-paced life, a poor diet and a deficiency of minerals and vitamins. Addressing your sleep quality and making it a priority is one of several key steps to climbing the ladder of health, wellness and external radiance and beauty.

So what is the definition of a good night's sleep and how can it be achieved? A good night's sleep can be defined as one that is uninterrupted and allows the body to cycle through all five sleep cycles.

The first four cycles of sleep are called non-REM sleep and include three cycles of light sleep, followed by the fourth cycle of very deep sleep. The fifth cycle is called REM sleep (rapid eye movement) where the brain is very active and dreaming occurs. A deficiency of REM sleep has been linked to mood disorders, depression, anxiety and irritability. The five cycles of sleep are approximately 90 to 110 minutes long and occur five to six times per night. Various factors such as age, caffeine intake, a poor diet, menopause, sleep medications, stress and bright lights from an alarm clock, television or window can interrupt the five cycles of sleep, leaving us in a state of mild to severe sleep deprivation. Without a constant rhythm of sleeping well and deeply, attempting to achieve health and beauty goals is often an exercise in futility.

Fatigue is involved in one out of every six vehicle accidents.

SLEEP AND WEIGHT LOSS

Studies indicate that if you sleep more, you will weigh less. In a recent study, researchers in Chicago identified two hormones, *leptin* and *ghrelin*, as having an influence on appetite, fat storage and cravings. Ghrelin, which is produced in the gastrointestinal tract, stimulates appetite, while leptin, produced in fat cells, sends a signal to the brain when you are full. When you don't get enough quality sleep, leptin levels drop, which means you don't feel as satisfied after you eat. Lack of sleep also causes ghrelin levels to rise, which means your appetite is stimulated and you want more food. These two factors combined can set the stage for overeating and cravings. In fact, the study also found that when leptin levels dropped due to sleep deprivation, the subject's desire for high carbohydrate- and calorie-dense food rose by a whopping 45 percent! I am by no means suggesting you give up exercise and eating well to sleep the day away in order to achieve your weight loss goals. However, I do recommend making your sleeping patterns a priority to boost your immune system, keep your hormonal system in check and lose or maintain your desired body weight.

> Some studies suggest women need up to an hour's extra sleep a night compared to men. For women, not getting enough restful sleep appears to be one reason women are much more susceptible to depression than men.

ACHIEVING QUALITY SLEEP

To achieve a proper amount of quality sleep, it is best to start implementing a nighttime pattern. Like most other areas of life, our systems respond best when they get into a routine. Although there will be times and stressors in your life that knock you off your sleep routine, try to implement the following sleep habits into your life to help establish a healing and well-rested sleep pattern.

1. Do not have a caffeinated beverage such as coffee, tea, pop/soda or green tea five hours or less prior to bedtime.

2. Do not eat high Glycemic Index foods prior to bedtime. These include white bread, pasta, bagels, white sugar, candy, chocolate, pop, coffee, granola bars, pretzels, cookies and cake.

3. If you must eat in the evening, try to select a protein source or a low Glycemic Index carbohydrate such as celery or cucumbers.

4. Keep your room as dark as possible. Any light in the room can upset melatonin release. Melatonin, a powerful anti-cancer hormone, is secreted in complete darkness from the pineal gland, typically from 2 a.m. to 4 a.m. If there is any light in the bedroom (from the bathroom, outside street lights or your alarm clock), it can interfere with melatonin secretion. If you must use a digital alarm clock, turn it away from the bed and invest in some pull-down blinds to make your room as dark as possible. Sleep masks can also work to help you sleep in complete darkness.

5. Avoid shift work whenever you can. It is impossible to have proper melatonin release while you are working a nighttime shift.

6. If you feel anxious about sleeping or suffer from insomnia, try putting lavender on your pillow cases or sheets. Lavender's aroma is relaxing and will help you ease into a peaceful slumber.

7. Do not smoke. In addition to being one of the biggest aging elements to your skin and loading your body with free radicals, smoking can also upset sleep patterns.

8. Do not watch the news or read the newspaper prior to bed. On an unconscious level, the images can imprint on your brain and psyche and cause a disrupted sleep pattern.

9. Once in bed, record in a journal your day's events and the things for which you are grateful. It is not enough to just think of your gratitudes; you must write them down. In a mysterious and unexplainable way, just writing down your thoughts, goals or most personal dreams has a calming and peaceful effect on the mind.

10. Avoid over-the-counter or prescribed sleep medica-

tions whenever you can. Sleep medications have been shown to reduce and upset the amount of REM sleep you get. A deficiency in REM sleep has been linked to several mood disorders such as depression and anxiety. If all else fails, try natural sleep aids such as valerian root (available at health food stores), time-released melatonin or chamomile tea.

11. Eat foods high in *tryptophan* and calcium to help you get to sleep. Tryptophan is a precursor to the brain chemical serotonin, which triggers proper melatonin release. Melatonin has been called the body's natural sleep aid. Low levels of melatonin are linked with insomnia and other sleep disturbances. Calcium has a calming and relaxing effect to help you ease into a proper and deep night's sleep. Tryptophan-rich foods include whole grains, turkey and dairy products.

12. Go to sleep and rise at the same time every day. Do not sleep in on weekends; this will only upset the routine you are trying to establish. Ideally, do not go to sleep later than 10 p.m.

13. Do not drink alcohol before bed.

Health Optimizer #2 — Engage in Compressive and Expansive Exercises Five Days Per Week

It is no secret that exercise is a critical component to achieving a healthy lifestyle. In addition to a nutrition-filled diet, physical fitness is the other major component that can prevent and reverse numerous disease processes such as heart disease, obesity, depression, stroke, insomnia, osteoporosis and fatigue.

In order to reap the most benefits from your exercise program, it is vital to include a compressive and expansive component of exercise into your schedule five times per week. Fear not. This does not mean you have to fit in a gym visit for an hour and a half each day while you are already struggling to balance your busy schedule. In fact, your entire exercise routine can be done in the comfort of your own home in 30 minutes a day, five times per week. Your total and complete physical fitness program should include both compressive and expansive exercises.

COMPRESSIVE EXERCISES

Compressive exercises put force onto your spine and bones while also including a cardiovascular component. Think of this type of exercise as a type of (compressive) pressure that strengthens and builds more bone, increasing the amount of calories burned while strengthening your heart and lungs. Examples of compressive exercises are weight training, fast walking, jumping, racquet sports, running and high-impact aerobics.

In order to maximize results, you should incorporate a weight-training session into your exercise schedule two to three times per week. A weight-training session does not need to last longer than 10 to 15 minutes for two body parts (i.e. arms and back). In terms of training, the body can be broken into upper body and lower body. Upper body parts are:

Chest—An example exercise to strengthen chest muscles is a push-up. To perform properly, place your hands on the floor slightly wider than your shoulders. Either on your knees or your toes, slowly bend arms and lower body until elbows are at 90 degree angles. Straighten arms and push up without locking elbows. Keep your abdominal muscles tight throughout the movement and avoid sagging in the middle!

Back—An example exercise for your back is a back extension. Lie flat on your stomach on the floor. Place hands behind your head or clasp them behind your back and slowly lift your chest off the floor a few inches. Hold for 10-15 seconds and release.

Shoulders—An example exercise for your shoulders is an overhead press. With your free weights, stand or sit with your feet shoulder width apart. Start with weight at eye level, hands wider than shoulders and arms at 90-degree angles. Slowly push the weight over your head (keep the weight slightly forward in front of your head so you can see it out of the corner of your eye) and lower back until elbows are at 90-degree angles. If you have neck or lower back problems, do the shoulder lift exercise instead of an overhead press.

Bicep—An example exercise to strengthen biceps is a concentration curl. Kneel on the floor or sit on a bench and grasp a dumbbell. Place the back of the upper arm on the inner thigh and lean into the leg to raise the elbow a bit. Raise your desired weight to front of shoulder and then lower until arm is almost fully extended.

Triceps—An example exercise to strengthen triceps is a kickback. Hold a weight in each hand and bend over until torso is parallel to the floor. Make sure your abdominal muscles are tight and legs are bent to take the strain off the lower back. Bend elbows and pull them even with back. Straighten arms behind you, squeezing the triceps and slowly lower back down.

Lower body parts for training are:

Legs—An example of an exercise to strengthen your leg muscles is to lunge with body weights. Position your feet shoulder width apart, with your feet pointing straight ahead. Pick up a pair of light weights (beginners may want to try without weights at first) bending at your knees to make sure you don't strain your back. To begin, step your right foot forward, keeping your forward leg centered over your ankle. Make sure your knee doesn't go beyond your toes. When coming back to the starting position (standing upright with knees slightly bent), focus on straightening your knee and hip. Think of your back leg as the balancer and your front leg as the mover. Switch and try with left leg.

Gluteal region (buttocks)—An example of an exercise to strengthen the gluteal area is a buttock lift. Lying on the floor, place your feet on top of a chair and a pillow under your neck to avoid hyperextension. Place the palms of your hands flat on the floor by your side. Exhale and contract your lower back and gluteal (buttock) region while you slightly raise up in a contraction (i.e., lifting buttock towards the ceiling). Hold for 3–5 seconds and slowly exhale and relax.

Abdominal musculature—An example of an exercise to strengthen the abdominal muscles is a reverse curl. The reverse curl targets the lower fibers of your abdominal muscles. Lie on your back and bend your knees towards your chest as far as is comfortable. Make sure to keep your hips on the floor. Contract your abdominal muscles to bring knees towards chest instead of swinging up legs with momentum. Exhale and slowly bring feet back to floor.

If you do not have a gym membership, simply purchase some free weights and/or exercise tubing to use at home. Exercise tubing and weights are typically labeled as light, medium or heavy. Select a resistance that is challenging but not impossible for you to work with. The key is to use a weight (or tension on elastic tubing) that feels fairly heavy and that you cannot lift easily over and over again. The duration of each set should include eight to 12 repetitions with two to three sets for each exercise. Once you can do 12 repetitions quite easily, increase the weight by 10 percent. There are many different types of weight-training options to tighten and tone your musculature. The table of the five-day sample exercise regime (table 7.1) targets all the main components of arms, legs, shoulder, chest and back. Once you have mastered these exercises, be sure to either increase your weight or switch to other weight-training options to ensure your muscles continue to be challenged. While doing weight-bearing exercises, it is important to maintain proper form, isolating the muscle being used. Take notice of the muscle you are working out and make sure that other surrounding and stronger musculature are not compensating for the exercise. I am also a huge advocate of learning as much as you can and visiting an expert in the field. I highly recommend investing in a personal trainer from time to time to ensure your form and technique is proper.

At rest, the heart beats between 60 to 100 times per minute.

Cardiovascular exercise such as fast walking, jogging, skipping, biking, running or using a treadmill should be done three times per week for a minimum of 20 minutes. My motto is "work harder, not longer." You should feel slightly out of breath while exercising, but still be able to hold a conversation if necessary. If you do not sweat or increase your heart rate past 20 to 25 beats per 10 seconds, I would recommend increasing your intensity and speed. Cardiovascular exercise can also be done in spurts to increase cardiovascular strength and caloric expenditure such as taking the stairs at work, parking in a distant parking spot and walking to the store. If your budget allows, invest in a stationary bicycle or treadmill for when the weather does not permit outdoor activity. Doing your cardiovascular workouts in the morning is always the best approach to boosting metabolic function. If you still have trouble finding time in your day to work out, set your alarm clock half an hour earlier for an early-morning walk, cycle, jog or run.

I recommend doing all of your compressive exercise (cardiovascular and a weight-training session) on the same day. See table 7.1 for a sample five-day exercise regime.

> Muscle is more metabolically active than fat. Individuals with more muscle mass have a higher resting metabolic rate and are usually leaner.

EXPANSIVE EXERCISES

In contrast to compressive exercises that put significant and necessary force on the bones, joints, ligaments and tendons in the body, expansive exercises open up and elongate the spine and musculature. These types of exercises improve posture, flexibility, breathing, quality of sleep and balance as well as reduce tension and blood pressure and strengthen the inner abdominal musculature (core strength). Both types of exercise (compressive and expansive) are equally important and serve to balance each other. Examples of expansive exercise are:

- **Yoga** There are many different styles of yoga to choose from, depending on your personality. They include Hatha yoga (gentle yoga), Ashtanga yoga (fast-paced, intense yoga), Kundalini yoga (focuses on the breath) and Bikram yoga, or "hot" yoga (practiced in a 95- to 100-degree Fahrenheit room). All yoga styles include the same postures with different emphasis on intensity, breathing and pace.

- **Pilates** This is a system of physical exercises invented in the 1920s by Joseph H. Pilates. This form of exercise involves controlled movements, stretching and breathing that builds core strength but does not build bulk. In addition to flexibility and balance, the Pilates series of movements engages both mind and body.

- **Tai chi** This is a form of martial art that focuses on cultivating the flow of energy in the body. Tai chi is done by performing slow, gentle and precise sequences of movements, called forms. The forms are done in double-stance and single-stance maneuvers in slow motion and involve flexion of musculature and extreme focus of the mind.

- **Morning stretches** After a night's sleep of inactivity, stretching out the muscles of the neck, back, legs, arms and shoulders will help to increase blood flow to these areas and relax your muscles. Incorporating morning stretches, for instance, in the shower, not only gets the blood flowing—it is wonderful for improving energy and digestion.

If you are new to expansive exercise, you should note that there is a learning curve. This form of exercise includes both mental and physical focus, meditation, patience and practice. It can take years for people to master the art of yoga, Pilates or tai chi. That said, the improvement of energy, breathing and postural changes that you will notice soon after engaging in this type of movement is unmatched by any other form of exercise.

If your time and budget permits, visit a class or studio or book a one-on-one session for any of the above-mentioned expansive exercises. If this is not feasible, there are several excellent home DVDs or videos that are specifically targeted for fast, easy and effective expansive training sessions.

Table 7.1: Sample Five-Day Exercise Regime

Monday	Tuesday	Wednes-day	Thursday	Friday	Saturday	Sunday
Compressive exercise day (arms and back)	Expansive exercise day	Compressive exercise day (shoulders and legs)	Rest	Compressive exercise day (arms and chest)	Rest	Expansive exercise day
Arms: Bicep curls Back: Front seated row	30-minute Pilates tape	Legs: Tubing squats and wall sits Shoulders: Weighted arm lifts to side and front		Arms: Triceps with dumb-bells Chest: Push-ups or chest press		30-minute Hatha yoga tape
20 minutes on the treadmill with incline		25-minute high-impact walk outside		20 minutes of intense cycling		

Monday	Tuesday	Wednes-day	Thursday	Friday	Saturday	Sunday
Stomach crunches (front and side crunches to target all sur-rounding abdominal muscula-ture)		Stomach crunches (front and side crunches to target all sur-rounding abdominal muscula-ture)		Stomach crunches (front and side crunches to target all sur-rounding abdomi-nal mus-culature)		

EASY-TO-DO COMPRESSIVE EXERCISES

Bicep Curls: Grab free weights or a weighted object with an underhand grip. Stand with your feet shoulder width apart. Keep your elbows close to your torso at all times. Moving only your forearms, use your bicep strength to curl the weight up to shoulder level. Hold this position for a second to maximize the peak contraction in the biceps. Slowly lower the weight to the starting position. Repeat three sets of 10 to 15 repetitions.

Figure 7.1: Bicep Curls

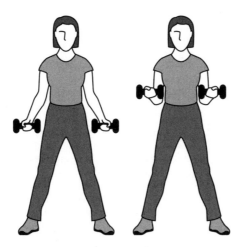

Front Seated Row: This exercise works the upper back and shoulders. Sit on the floor with your legs extended and your knees slightly bent. Place exercise tubing around the arch of both feet and hold the handles or ends in each hand. Sit up tall with your palms facing the floor and your arms extended in front, slightly lower than shoulder height. Bend your elbows and pull the tubing towards you while squeezing your shoulder blades together. Make sure to sit upright and pull your tummy in tight.

Figure 7.2: Front Seated Row

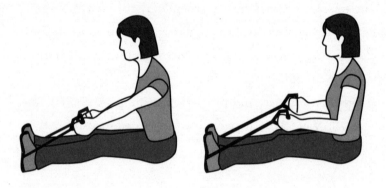

Tubing Squats: This exercise tightens the musculature in the buttocks area. Hold one handle of the tubing in each hand and step onto the tubing. Your feet should be in line with your hips. Shift your weight to your heels, bend the knees and pretend to sit down in a chair. While in the squatting position, pull the tubing tight by wrapping it once gently around each hand. Push from your heels and straighten up into a standing position. Repeat three sets of squats with 15 repetitions each.

Figure 7.3: Tubing Squats

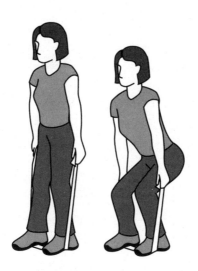

Wall Sits: Lean against a wall with your feet placed shoulder width apart. Slowly lower your body until your upper thighs are parallel to the floor or your knees are bent at a 90-degree angle. Hold the position for the desired amount of time (e.g., 30 seconds working up to two minutes). Position your feet far enough from the wall that your knees do not go past your toes when you are in the lowest position; overextending may lead to knee pain or injury. Keep your upper back and shoulders against the wall and cross your arms in front of your chest. This movement is most challenging at the bottom of the motion when your knees are bent at 90 degrees. If this is too difficult, only go down halfway until you are ready for the full range of motion.

Figure 7.4: Wall Sits

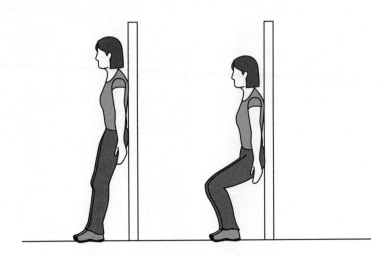

Shoulder Lifts: Stand with your feet shoulder width apart and your arms by your side. Grab a weight in each hand and raise your arms out from your sides with your palms facing upward, until your arms are level with your shoulders. Once you have raised your arms to shoulder height, turn your palms down and slowly lower the weight. This exercise can also be done lifting your arms with weights straight in front of your body. Repeat for three sets of 10 to 15 presses.

Figure 7.5: Shoulder Lifts

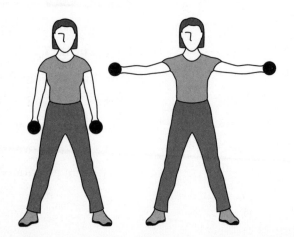

Triceps with Dumbbells: Sit on a flat bench or your bed with your feet flat on the floor. Grasp the dumbbell in one hand with an overhand grip (palm facing forward). Extend your arm fully up, and hold the dumbbell over your head. Try to keep your elbow as close to your body as possible. As you extend your elbow, fully contract your triceps and hold the extension at the top of the movement. If you find you are overextending your lower back during this exercise, it is an indication that the dumbbell is too heavy. Begin with a 5-pound weight and move up from there. Repeat three sets of 10 to 15 repetitions.

Figure 7.6: Triceps with Dumbbells

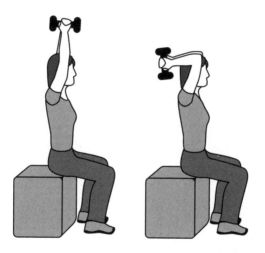

Chest Presses: Lie on your back with your knees bent and your feet flat on the floor. Hold the weights (5, 7, 10 pounds or more) in each hand with your arms extended out from your body like a cross. Bend your arms at the elbows towards the ceiling. Exhale as you push up towards the ceiling. Hold for a count of three and inhale as you bring the weight back to the starting position. Repeat for three sets of 10 to 15 presses.

Figure 7.7: Chest Presses

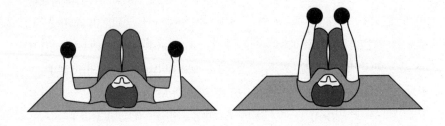

Health Optimizer #3 — Get Happy!

"Most people are about as happy as they make up their minds to be."
—Abraham Lincoln

Happiness is a very personal and subjective feeling. What makes one person happy may not make another feel joy. For instance, staying home and hunkering down with your family at night may bring you great personal satisfaction, while another person may thrive on being a socialite and going from party to party. Is the full-time mom who loves being with her children any happier than the successful business executive who gets a thrill out of putting together business ventures? Not necessarily. The happiness of others is not for us to judge, as it is incredibly different from person to person. The key is to focus on your joy and what truly "floats your boat." Is it painting? Cooking? Having more free time? Perhaps you would like to become a proficient gardener? As your third and final health optimizer, personal happiness, or lack of it, is a critical factor in your overall state of wellness. In addition to reaping the benefits of doing a nutritional makeover, it is equally important to do an emotional makeover from time to time.

MIND AND BODY

The powerful and unmistakable connection between the mind and body has gained a lot more attention and research dollars in the past few decades. In fact, an entire field of medicine called *psychoneuroimmunology* is now dedicated to this connection. Psychoneuroimmunology is a field of medicine that addresses the effects of psychology (thoughts) and neurology (brain and nervous system) on the immune system. Hundreds of studies done in this area suggest that anxiety and stress can weaken immune system responses and make people more vulnerable to certain diseases. Likewise, positive emotional states appear to help strengthen immune system responses. This connection is the reason why some people fall ill after a personal tragedy, an intense exam period or a family trauma such as divorce. This is also why your state of mind is one of the greatest predictors of your inner health and therefore your outer beauty. Unfortunately, people are more stressed today than ever before. Perhaps this is from higher job and family demands, the faster pace of life, the cost of living, or the lack of minerals, essential fats and vitamins in their diets. Whatever the reasons, depressive disorders are on the rise with about 10 percent to 20 percent of the population diagnosed with a mild to moderate form of depression. As it stands, depressive disorders are the second leading cause of disability in North America, and women are diagnosed two times as often as men.

> The risk of a heart attack appears to triple within an hour of driving in traffic.

To tap into your own source of happiness, I draw on Shakespeare's famous quote, "This above all—to thine own self be true." The only path to true happiness is to be true to yourself. Completely eliminating stress from your life is not possible or realistic. As sure as Christmas will come every year, stressors will always pop up and push your buttons. Some stressors will be minor, such as losing your wallet, while others, such as losing a loved one, will literally take your breath away (and may they be few and far between). The goal is not to get rid of life's constant challenges; it is to enjoy, enhance and even heal your state of mind so you can endure the constant bumps without being thrown off course.

> Depression is reported to cost U.S. employers $44 billion per year in lost productivity.

In order to discover how to be true to yourself, sit calmly in a quiet room and answer the following questions:

1. If I were to win the lottery, I would: _____

   _____

   _____

   _____ .

2. If I were to win the lottery, I would stop: _____

   _____

   _____

   _____ .

3. I feel the happiest and most peaceful when: _____

   _____

   _____

   _____ .

4.   I feel the most stressed when: _____

_____

_____

_____ .

5.   The part of me I would like to change most is: _____

_____

_____

_____ .

By answering these questions, you will zero in on a constant theme. Everyone has a different area of life that causes her the greatest turmoil. It may be related to finances, spirituality, relationships, family or vocation. Try to notice which area causes you the most anxiety and lost sleep. Perhaps if you won the lottery, you would start an interior design business, write children's books or spend more time at home. Also pay attention to when and where you feel most tense. Is it at the office? At home? In the car? Once you have identified your sources of stress, taking quantifiable "baby steps" to improve your happiness will reduce your anxiety and stress. What are quantifiable steps? They are steps that are specific to you, accountable and achievable within a realistic period of time. For example, if your greatest stressor is not having enough money, your quantifiable baby steps may be:

1.   I will stop buying a specialty coffee every morning and make coffee at home. I will save the difference ($4 per day, $28 per week, $112 per month, $5,824 per year!) in a separate account for "rainy days."

2.   I will affirm thoughts of abundance daily. I will say in my head upon awakening and going to sleep, "I attract abundance and money into my life." Remember, your thoughts will become your reality!

3. I will write down the amount of money I would like to make per year and devise a business plan in the next two weeks for how to generate or save it, e.g., switching jobs, getting a second job, cutting luxury costs such as dining out, having a garage sale, not buying new clothes, etc.

Even if the steps forward appear to be too small or too insignificant to make a difference, they are not. Once you take action towards your definition of happiness, it will have a domino and cumulative effect that will result in a slow (or sometimes fast) movement towards your innermost desires. Commit to taking these steps and you will soon notice how quickly you are propelled to where you want to be. In addition to taking quantifiable baby steps, it is also critical to have a "joy factor" in your life that is just for you. Commit to treating yourself once a day or week with something that allows you a little breather. Finding your joy factor does not have to be costly; it can be something as simple as meditating, going for a walk or planting some flowers. Fill in the following statements in order to pinpoint your joy factor:

1. In order to feel better about myself I will: _____

_____

_____

_____

by (insert date) _____
(Whatever your pleasure—just go for it! It could be losing 20 pounds, updating your wardrobe, buying yourself flowers, going for a manicure, pedicure or massage, whatever—you deserve it!)

2. One way I will reduce stress in my life is to_____

_____

_____

(e.g., buy a yoga tape, take a half hour a day by yourself, stretch, listen to music)

3.   I will start doing _____

_____

to move towards my greatest joy and passion.

THE HAPPY FORMULA

The definition of happiness is different for everyone. Although our definition of happiness differs, the path to getting there is based on the same formula that, when followed, works! The specifics involved in the happy formula are:

Keep a journal. Keep a journal by your bedside to write in nightly. Record your thoughts in two categories: 1) Things I am grateful for and 2) Goals. Writing down a minimum of five things you are grateful for nightly will keep you in an abundant and positive frame of mind. When writing your goals, break them down into daily, weekly, monthly and yearly aspirations. Be sure to put a time frame on your goals so you can look back and assess your progress. To be even more specific, when setting goals, divide them into the following four areas of life: personal, professional, financial and spiritual. It is not enough to just think about your goals; you need to write them down and commit them to paper.

Take action steps. Once you have set your goals and written them down, you have planted the seed of intention. Although setting your goals is the most critical step, you need an action plan in order to see your goals come to fruition. For example, if your goal is to improve the look and feel of your skin, start implementing action steps in that direction, such as supplementing with fish oils, following the five-day cleanse outlined in chapter 3 and eating raw fruits and vegetables. Although I would love to tell you that once you set a goal, your innermost desires will fall from the sky, you already know that for most of us this does not happen. Goals are achieved by setting your intentions down on paper and taking constant action steps towards your dreams. Without taking the necessary steps, it is like putting gas into your car without turning on the engine. The good news is that this formula works for everyone. Before you know it, through intentions and actions, all of your heart's desires will become reality.

Read inspiring literature. It is important to learn from the great minds of the past and present. These are the people who have had goals, set them, and taken action steps to achieve their dreams. Luckily, all you have to do in order to tap into the minds of great thinkers and writers is to visit your local bookstore or library. Your mind (both conscious and unconscious) is similar to a sponge and will take in all the information you feed it, good or bad. This is why it is so important to be very specific and selective about the material you allow into your mind. Watching mindless reality TV all night long will not get you closer to your dreams and goals. Although watching movies and occasional television shows is a reality for most of us, I highly recommend taking the time to read inspirational and motivational books daily. It does not matter if it is only for 15 minutes a day; the key is to expose your mind to "food for the soul." A few starter books to get you on your way are *The Alchemist* by Paulo Coelho, *The Four Agreements* by Don Miguel Ruiz, *Wherever You Go There You Are* by Jon Kabat-Zinn. Other authors whose work I recommend are Wayne Dyer, Deepak Chopra, Robin Sharma and Gary Zukav.

Meditate. When most people think of meditating, an image of a man sitting in a white robe with incense burning beside him is conjured up in their minds. This is definitely not the type of meditating to which I am referring. Similar to happiness, meditation is very personal and specific. The role of meditating is to clear your mind from all cluttering thoughts and to be still and quiet for a specific amount of time each day. By doing so, in an unexplainable way, you will find yourself better equipped to deal with your daily stressors, more aware of the opportunities or signs that pop up in your life and more in tune with your inner self. In today's "go, go, go" society, most people feel stressed at the thought of taking a mental break even for a short time. Remember, your body and mind craves a certain period of daily meditation in order to be at the top of your game—physically, mentally and emotionally. Similar to developing a muscle, your "meditation muscle" will strengthen over time. So how do you begin? Simply find a 15-minute block of time (ideally first thing in the morning) to sit alone (on a cushion on the floor with legs crossed or in a chair) and breathe. Start by focusing on long inhales through your nose and long exhales through your nose. Focus on your belly rising and falling. Most of us breathe with the upper chest during times of stress, so be sure that your breath is coming from your lower belly region. When first beginning, your mind will likely wander off to invading thoughts such as what you have packed the kids for lunch or what you need to get done at the office. Do not stop your 15-minute session; simply and gently bring your mind back to the focus of your breath. If your mind still has a difficult time settling down, start by focusing on one word with your inhale (for instance, think of the word "peace") and exhale (think of a word to describe what you would like to be rid of, such as the word "stress"). Alternatively, keep shifting your focus to a constant image such as a burning candle.

Eat well and exercise. As author Adelle Davis so eloquently wrote, "We are indeed much more than what we eat, but what we eat can nevertheless help us to be much more than what we are." This entire book has been dedicated to achieving inner health with food and supplements so our beauty and radiance can shine through. As you have likely discovered by reading the previous chapters and changing your diet, your nutritional choices affect your chemistry, which in turn affects your mood, body weight and appearance. Of course your food choices do not determine your entire state of happiness, but as the most powerful influence over brain chemistry, nutrition plays a fundamental role. In addition to diet, exercise will release feel-good chemicals called endorphins that also contribute to your mood and overall emotional well-being.

You have just finished reading all the information you need to propel you up the ladder of optimal health to reveal the most beautiful, vibrant you! Chapter 8 will answer additional questions you may have about your health and beauty. It's followed by delicious and easy-to-make recipes. Enjoy!

chapter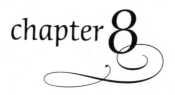

COMMON QUESTIONS ANSWERED

"To eat is a necessity, but to eat intelligently is an art."

—LA ROCHEFOUCAULD

When it comes to the world of nutrition, I have found there are two truths:

1. Nutrition is very personal.
2. Everyone is an expert.

While I encourage everyone to become educated and active participants in their health, there are many misunderstandings that exist about nutrition. These misunderstandings are partially created by fad diets, difficulty interpreting tricky labeling and trendy media stories that hit our daily news. Finding out the truths behind confusing nutritional messages is often difficult and far too time consuming. In an attempt to clear up any food misnomers or dieting confusion that may exist in your mind, this chapter has the answers to your need-to-know questions. From the safety of soy and trans fats, to the old debate about butter versus margarine, it's time to get down to the facts! If you have a question that has not been answered by the following section or the information outlined in this book, I would like to hear from you! Simply visit my website and email your questions to www.drjoey.com.

I have tried every diet and cannot lose weight. Is it possible to increase my metabolism?

Atkins, South Beach, Weight Watchers … Do any of these diets sound familiar to you? Millions of North Americans are on a diet, and yet 67 percent of the population is overweight or obese. How can that be? In truth, a lot of the popular diets on the market today are not sensible or sustainable for long periods of time. Whether it is drastically reducing carbohydrates and increasing proteins and saturated fat foods such as advocated by extreme Atkins devotees, or counting points that relate to food as in Weight Watchers, it appears for some, the results are not long lasting.

As in any area of life, including healthcare, knowledge is power. Once you understand the "why" behind eating certain foods such as low Glycemic Index carbohydrates, lean proteins and essential fats, healthy eating does not have to be a temporary "fad," "program" or "diet." When you approach nutrition from a knowledge base, healthy eating and achieving your desired weight will last a lifetime. This is where the Pick-3 System of eating discussed in chapter 4 applies. By combining proteins, fats and carbohydrates at every meal and snack, your blood sugar and insulin levels will remain balanced, resulting in weight loss, endless energy and prevention against future disease and illness.

In my last book, *The Metabolism Boosting Diet*, I detailed a specific plan for getting you to your goal weight. My entire career has been dedicated to health and weight loss. What I know for sure is that the way to lose weight, make peace with food and feel your very best naturally is through hormonal weight loss (also known as blood sugar control). The Pick-3 System of eating is based on hormonal weight loss. This system of eating will keep you satisfied and in blood sugar balance so you feel great and hit your target weight. In addition to the recipes outlined in this book, if you would like a more detailed plan, simply pick up a copy of *The Metabolism Boosting Diet* to learn more. Now ... let's learn a little bit more about the concept of metabolism.

When it comes to dieting and weight loss, the concept of metabolism is often referred to. Metabolism is the amount of calories you burn at rest, or the amount of energy your body uses to function.

The average 30-year-old woman burns approximately 1150 to 1250 calories daily, while the average 30-year-old man uses 1600 calories. After age 30, metabolism slows down and drops about one-half of a percent each year. This may not seem like a lot, but it adds up. This is why, as we age, we either have to exercise more or eat wiser in order to avoid the battle of the bulge. In addition to age, chronic yo-yo dieting (gaining and losing weight continually) also slows down metabolism. Luckily, there are certain methods and activities that can jump-start your metabolism to make the pounds melt away. The following steps rev up your metabolic engine and facilitate weight loss.

1. Increase your protein consumption for an eight-week period. By doing so, you will release more of the hormone *glucagon* (insulin's opposite), which facilitates fat loss. However, this does not mean that you should exclude carbohydrates. On the contrary, your body will need to eat low Glycemic Index carbohydrates in the form of vegetables, (most) fruits and a modest amount of whole grains. Increasing your protein consumption at each meal will help get the weight loss ball rolling. I recommend having an approximate 1:1 protein to carbohydrate ratio for an eight-week period. For instance, if you're eating 20 grams of protein, then consume 20 grams of carbohydrates.

2. Drink three cups of green tea daily. Green tea increases metabolic rate and speeds up fat oxidation. Compounds in green tea speed up the rate at which calories are burned and therefore increase overall energy expenditure, and this in turn leads to weight loss.

3. Supplement with metabolism-boosting ingredients such as chromium (a trace mineral), conjugated linoleic

acid (a fatty acid) and green tea extract (epigallocate-
chin gallate, or EGCG). Their benefits are:

Green Tea Extract

- Contains powerful antioxidants called catechin
  polyphenols that help fight free radicals in the
  body that cause disease, aging and weight retention

- Helps to burn belly fat

- Helps to burn more calories

- Boosts metabolic capacity

Conjugated Linoleic Acid (CLA)

- Increases lean muscle mass and accelerates fat
  loss

- Increases metabolic rate

- Protects against fat gain following weight loss (in
  other words—helps you to keep the weight off!)

Chromium

- Monitors blood sugar

- Aids metabolism

- Reduces food cravings

Please visit www.drjoey.com to learn more.

4. Investigate the possibility of food allergies or sensitivities. Foods that you react to tend to cause your body to
   cling to excess fat, which makes weight loss extremely
   difficult. The most common food sensitivities include
   dairy, wheat, gluten and soy. If, after you have done
   the five-day cleanse outlined in chapter 3 and after
   following the Pick-3 System of eating for a minimum
   of two to four weeks, you do not lose weight, you
   should investigate the possibility of food sensitivities
   or hormonal imbalances (i.e., sluggish thyroid or elevated cortisol levels). Food-allergy testing can be done
   by following an elimination diet or by visiting a natural healthcare practitioner. Elimination diets involve

completely eliminating the suspected food irritant for a three-week period. Following this period, introduce the suspected food, e.g., dairy or wheat, and monitor your symptoms. Hormonal testing can be done by your doctor via bloodwork.

5. Increase caloric expenditure by exercising. Pick your favorite activity and start moving. Although I have mentioned in previous chapters not to focus on calories, if you are at a metabolic standstill, you need to start moving and burning more to rev up your metabolic engine. The following table shows examples of the amount of calories burned through various exercises.

Table 8.1: Caloric Expenditure per Exercise

Activity	Number of Minutes	Calories Burned
Biking (moderate)	30	286
Jogging	30	250
Stationary bike	30	214
Swimming	30	286
Walking (less than 2 mph)	30	250
Weight lifting	30	125
Yoga	30	143

I find my skin is quite dry and I am developing wrinkles. What can I do?

In an attempt to clear up dry skin and prevent wrinkles, women are slathering their bodies with the latest anti-aging moisturizing creams. Although moisturizers can be very helpful in improving the look and feel of your skin, the other key to decreasing fine lines and improving your complexion is to decrease free radical damage from occurring at a rapid rate.

A majority of fancily packaged skin care products on the market today contain various toxins that will be absorbed by your skin. In fact, it is currently estimated that more than 8 percent of all the cosmetic products currently contain one or more ingredients that have been documented to cause adverse reactions. Because the layers of your skin act like a strainer, harmful synthetic substances such as moisturizing creams penetrate and pass right into your body. If you are using a product daily, it's best to know which type of cream is safest to use. When purchasing creams or moisturizers for your face and body:

- Avoid products that contain synthetic fragrances and dyes that may aggravate your already pre-existing skin condition.
- Be wary of toners that contain alcohol. Alcohol-based toners disturb the pH level of your skin leaving it much drier than it was in the first place.
- Visit your local health food store and inquire about natural skin care products with essential oils and antioxidants such as *alpha lipoic acid, co-enzyme Q10, L-carnitine,* vitamin E, *retinol,* grapeseed oil, avocado oil or soybean oil.
- Investigate creams that contain *hyaluronic acid* (HA). Although they are more costly, these provide structural support to the skin, while retaining its moisture. HA has been shown to be very effective in reducing wrinkles and treating burns, surgical incisions and skin lesions.

As skin is the largest organ in your body, its condition is often a reflection of internal health rather than the result of external skin care products or irritants such as soaps and detergents. Premature wrinkling, dry skin, roughness, eczema, rosacea and acne are all reflections that our inner health is "off."

As we age, our skin tends to change as the body produces less oil, leaving our skin rough and dry. In addition, in the deeper layers of our skin, a decrease of two proteins called collagen and elastin cause the skin to thin, wrinkle and sag. Although the integrity of your skin is partially influenced by hereditary factors, other factors such as sunlight, smoking, eating inflammatory foods, harsh chemicals and stress can all accelerate the aging process. The most effective approach to ward off wrinkles and improve the look of your skin is to:

- Supplement with fish oils to get the benefits derived from the essential fat omega-3. Start with 2 to 3 grams daily of a high-quality fish oil in capsule form. Similar to the way a conditioner coats a hair follicle to make it shiny and smooth, the omega-3 fats found in fish oils add the necessary moisture to your skin, making it feel smoother and look younger.
- Investigate overall digestive health and potential food allergens as the cause of your dry or irritated skin.
- Increase your consumption of fruits and vegetables rich in *phytochemicals*. A recent study published in the *American Journal of Clinical Nutrition* (January 2005) concluded that consuming antioxidants from fruits and vegetables may decrease the oxidative stress that occurs during aging. Oxidative damage is partially responsible for wrinkles and sagging skin. Specifically vitamin

C and phytochemicals called *flavonoids*, found in green tea, soy and berries, promote the production of collagen and elastin—elements that keep skin looking youthful and vibrant.

- Do not smoke. Smoking ages the skin dramatically. I can usually spot a smoker's skin immediately.
- Do not overexpose yourself to the sun. A maximum of 20 minutes in the sun unprotected is plenty of time to get your vitamin D without doing damage.
- Reduce stress to decrease oxidative damage from occurring in your skin. Whether you practice meditation, journal, work out or pray, take steps to relax, breathe and "go with the flow" a little more.
- Avoid inflammatory foods such as sugar, trans fats and saturated fats found in red meats and full-fat cheeses.

I have continual bags and puffiness under my eyes. What can I do?

Simply looking at an individual's skin, hair, nails and eyes can often tell you a lot about her state of health. Like other symptoms in the body, swelling and puffiness under the eyes is often a clue that something else is "off." As you now know, the system that influences overall health the most is the digestive system. Whether you are experiencing eczema, bags under the eyes or bloating, it is important to investigate the health of your digestive system. Start by asking yourself the following questions:

- Do I have a regular bowel movement (once per day without strain)?

- Do I have cramping or diarrhea after I eat a certain food?
- Do I feel bloated all the time?

Clearing up digestive health by following the five-day cleanse outlined in chapter 3 will create the environment in which your health and beauty will flourish. In summary, the best way to optimize digestive health is:

1. Chew your food. By gulping down large particles of food, undigested food particles will end up in the gut. These food particles can be perceived as invaders and "attacked" by your immune system, thus creating many health problems.
2. Slow down your eating. It takes a minimum of 20 minutes for the brain to register a full signal from the digestive system.
3. Any time you are on an antibiotic, follow it up with a round of probiotics such as *acidophilus* and *bifidus*.
4. If you have chronic digestive problems, you may not be secreting the necessary digestive enzymes to properly break down your food. Visit your local health food store and inquire about an enzyme mix that will assist with digestion and absorption.
5. Make sure your diet contains plenty of fiber. Supplement with a minimum of 1 tablespoon of ground flaxseeds daily.
6. Stop eating a minimum of two hours prior to bedtime to give your body a daily mini cleanse and fast. This allows your digestive juices to burn up any residual waste in the gut.
7. Eliminate refined flours and sugars from your diet. In addition to causing weight gain, they can clog your system and cause bloating.

8. Drink six to eight glasses of fresh, clean water daily with lemon, a natural astringent.

Other common factors such as fluid retention, allergies, stress, medication and/or alcohol consumption can also cause dark circles and puffiness under the eyes. Allergic "shiners" or dark circles under the eyes may often be caused by a sensitivity or allergy to a protein in a food. Because cow's milk is far more protein-dense than human or goat's milk (15 percent versus 5 percent), cow's milk is the number one food sensitivity that you should suspect. I recommend removing dairy products completely from your diet for a three-week period to see if there are any significant changes. Other food sensitivities that should be eliminated on a one-by-one basis include wheat, soy, citrus, chocolate and gluten.

To soothe your eye area, lie down for 15 minutes a day with raw cucumber slices over each eye. Cool teabags or cotton wool pads soaked in witch hazel can also be quite soothing.

What is the difference between whole wheat and whole grain bread?

There is a lot of confusion for consumers when it comes to purchasing the right kind of bread. Most people equate brown bread with health, but this is not always true. Certain types of whole wheat bread are produced from refined and processed flour. The brown appearance of the bread is due to the addition of a small amount of blackstrap molasses or other browning agents. Similar to white refined bread, whole wheat bread from refined flour is higher on the Glycemic Index and will cause blood sugar and insulin levels to bounce around, which can result in fatigue and weight gain.

As soon as you complete your five-day cleanse, a certain amount of the right type of bread is included in your diet. The key is to eat whole grain bread, not refined whole wheat bread. Whole grain bread contains a higher fiber content, is loaded with minerals and vitamins, does not cause energy levels to fluctuate and keeps you feeling fuller longer. So ... how do you know if a loaf of bread is whole grain? Follow the steps below to make sure your bread passes the "bread test."

THE BREAD TEST

1. Check the ingredients label. Avoid food items that list "whole wheat," "enriched wheat flour" or "wheat flour." Instead, look for breads made with "100% whole wheat" or "whole grain."
2. Check the fiber content. You want to ensure a slice of bread has a minimum of 1.5 to 2 grams of fiber per slice. Most white refined breads contain approximately 0.5 grams of fiber per slice.
3. Do the "squeeze test." Most whole grain breads are denser due to their fiber content; they actually feel a little heavier. Whole grain breads cannot be squeezed into half their size, nor do they melt in your mouth like refined white breads do. Due to their higher fiber content, whole grain breads need to be chewed a little bit more.
4. Opt for sprouted-grain breads. When you eat a sprouted grain, you pre-digest the starch (carbohydrate content) and therefore lower the Glycemic Index response. In addition, sprouted-grain breads contain higher enzyme and mineral activity than refined, floury breads.
5. After you eat bread, notice if you feel tired soon after. Food items that are higher on the Glycemic Index often leave you in a hypoglycemic (low blood sugar)

and fatigued state. This is also the time that cravings for starch or sugar may kick in.

6. Do not be fooled by the words "fortified with." Fortification typically occurs with refined grains. Precious nutrients that have been stripped away during the refining process are added back in.

Start becoming familiar with less traditional grain items such as spelt, kamut, quinoa and almond flour. These types of foods can reduce cholesterol and high blood pressure and can even be beneficial in the prevention of heart disease, cancer, obesity and diabetes.

If you are opting to go gluten-free, please see the appendix for a list of gluten-free grains.

Is it okay to drink coffee?

Ah ... coffee. Who doesn't love the morning lift you get from your morning java? Coffee has become more than a drink—it has become part of our language and culture! We have all stood in line in one of the several hundred coffee shops that appear on our streets and heard the complicated orders: "I'll have a double, decaf, mocha, no whip, grande, light, no foam coffee, please." Indeed, coffee is so popular that our most trendy bookstores have merged with coffee chains such as Starbucks to make the book-buying experience even more pleasurable for consumers!

Even now, while I am sitting and writing about coffee's pros and cons, I am happily sipping away at my "one a day" indulgence (it's organic and sweetened with unrefined sugar)! Still, the pros and cons of coffee are hotly debated and must be considered. Let's begin with a discussion of the pros. Current research conducted at

Harvard University showed that regular coffee consumption lowered the risk of Type II diabetes. Why this is the case is unclear and further research into this area needs to be conducted. Other studies have shown that coffee may reduce the risk of developing gallstones, prevent the development of colon cancer and improve cognitive function.

But there is a downside to coffee. Coffee is highly acidic and can leach precious minerals from our systems. Remember, for optimal health and disease prevention, the goal is for the environment of our bodies to be more alkaline than acidic. Coffee can also cause anxiety, heart palpitations and raise blood pressure; it can also be highly addictive. Many report that drinking too much coffee can actually leave them feeling more tired than alert. Lastly, the diuretic effect of coffee must be taken into account by compensating with the consumption of water.

So … with all this information, do I give coffee a thumbs-up or a thumbs-down? I believe that one cup of coffee a day is safe to drink, as long as you are not pregnant and do not experience side effects from it such as the jitters or anxiety. I do recommend purchasing organic coffee, as nonorganic coffee beans are heavily sprayed with herbicides and pesticides. Although organic is more costly, it's well worth the investment. I also encourage coffee drinkers to avoid "coffee whiteners" that are loaded with partially hydrogenated fats. I am not convinced that drinking coffee will prevent or assist with Type II diabetes. I am eager to see more research in this area. Coffee can reduce sensitivity to insulin and tends to cause blood sugar levels to fluctuate (especially when sugar is added). The bottom line is that coffee should be a "treat," not a beverage to rely on for energy or hydration.

If you experience negative effects from coffee, or are looking for a wonderful and energy boosting replacement, try green tea for its antioxidant, fat-burning and energizing effects.

What is a safe sugar substitute?

The average North American consumes approximately 20 teaspoons of sugar per day. Common and inexpensive sugars such as high fructose corn syrup and sucrose (table sugar) are used in refined and low-fat food products to enhance taste and increase product sales. From soda pop, cookies and low-fat yogurt to ketchup and even some vitamins and toothpaste, sugar is a common health culprit that is widespread in our food sources. The ill effects of sugar on health are numerous. To name just a few, excess sugar intake results in excess weight gain, a decrease in energy levels, dental decay, suppression of immune system function and an increase in acidity. Because the public is becoming more aware of the ill effects of eating refined sugar, an alternative is now popping up in our grocery stores. Sugar substitutes are one of the largest-growing food products on the market. In fact, nearly 1,500 foods are sweetened with sugar substitutes and 144 million Americans use sugar substitutes on a regular basis. Yet, the question—are these sugar substitutes safe—needs to be addressed.

The Food and Drug Administration (FDA) has approved four sugar substitutes for use in a variety of foods: saccharin, aspartame, acesulfame-K, and sucralose. The commercial names for these types of sweeteners that appear on ingredients lists and in your grocery stores are:

- Saccharin = Sweet'n Low
- Aspartame = Nutrasweet or Equal

- Acesulfame potassium = Sunett or Sweet One
- Sucralose = Splenda

Saccharin and aspartame have both been the subject of ongoing controversy due to their links to potential health threats. Saccharin is the granddaddy of sweeteners and has been around since 1879. Controversy arose in the 1970s when rat studies showed that an overconsumption of saccharin could cause bladder cancer. Following those studies, saccharin carried a label that warned of its potential risk. In the year 2000, that label was removed, and saccharin is considered safe again by the Food and Drug Administration. Aspartame was first discovered by accident in 1965 by chemist James Schlatter while he was working on a peptic ulcer drug. This type of sweetener consists of three components: the amino acids *phenylalanine, aspartic acid* and *methanol,* otherwise known as wood alcohol. Methanol is toxic in humans even when consumed in small amounts. Although research studies have not yet been able to prove that aspartame causes neurological disorders, some of the most documented side effects include headaches, migraines, seizures, dizziness, muscle spasm, heart palpitations and numbness. If you suffer from a rare disease called *phenylketonuria,* you do not break down the amino acid phenylalanine and will not be able to consume aspartame even in small amounts.

Acesulfame potassium was approved by the FDA in 1998. This product is gaining more and more popularity and is currently used in thousands of food items. There are, however, claims that the FDA's approval of this product was based on flawed studies and that it indeed may cause cancer in animals.

I have my concerns regarding these three sweeteners. Although they are deemed safe by the FDA, I have witnessed both personal and professional accounts that report ill health symptoms that began with the onset of sweeteners such as aspartame and ceased when aspartame was removed from the diet. In the cases of aspartame, saccharin and acesulfame potassium, I wholeheartedly believe that they are best left out of our diets.

Sucralose, otherwise called Splenda, is the fourth and final artificial sweetener approved by the FDA. Splenda is created in the laboratory by chlorinating a sugar molecule. Over 100 animal studies have been conducted and indicate that Splenda appears to be safe for consumption. Studies done on humans are limited.

There are numerous natural sweeteners such as organic applesauce, apple butter, plum butter and mashed bananas and honey. Also, you can limit your sugar use by only using half the amount recommended in most recipes. You will be surprised how good your recipe tastes even with half the amount of sugar. Certain sweeter spices such as vanilla, ginger, cinnamon, nutmeg and orange can be added to baked goods to sweeten up a recipe. Sweetness from natural fruit in the form of berries (blueberries, raspberries and strawberries), apples and mangos are also a wonderful addition to any diet. Other natural sugar substitutes include:

> **Coconut sugar:** Coconut sugar is nutritious sugar and has a low score on the Glycemic Index, meaning you will not experience a blood sugar crash from it. I use this sugar option for baking, in tea, etc.

> **Brown rice syrup:** Gluten- and wheat-free, brown rice syrup is more suitable for cooking than adding to your tea. It has a slightly butterscotch flavor and can be used as a drizzle over healthy pancakes.

> **Honey:** Honey is chock-full of antioxidants and has been shown to be beneficial in lowering cholesterol. When selecting honey, remember that darker honey

has more nutrients and tends to be more flavorful. Substitute ½ cup of honey for every 1 cup of sugar.

Stevia: Made from a plant found in Paraguay, stevia is often used as a sweetener in tea, coffee or baked goods. Stevia is 200 to 300 times sweeter than sugar, so less is needed. Some brands of stevia have a slight "licorice" aftertaste, so experiment until you find one you like.

Applesauce: Applesauce is often used as a replacement for oil in baked goods. You can reduce the oil and/or butter in your recipe by half to three quarters and replace it with applesauce.

Maple syrup: Maple syrup is one of my favorite sweeteners to use for baking as it is naturally sweet and is an excellent source of manganese and a good source of zinc, which is important in maintaining a healthy immune system. To substitute maple syrup in your baking, you should use one third less maple syrup than the amount of sugar that is called for (i.e., ⅔ cup of maple syrup versus 1 cup of sugar). You should also decrease the wet ingredients by approximately 2 tablespoons for every ½ cup of maple syrup added.

SINLESS TRUFFLES

Makes 12 truffles

I love this recipe and often use it around the holiday season! These truffles are über-decadent ... and are filled to the brim with nutritional value.

Ingredients

½ cup pitted prunes

¼ cup pitted dates

3 tablespoons almond or cashew butter

1 tablespoon maple syrup

3 tablespoons unsweetened cocoa

½ cup finely grated unsweetened coconut

Directions

Drop pitted prunes and dates through the feed hole in a food processor one by one. Scrape the processor bowl and run until the prunes and dates are smooth. Add remaining ingredients except for the coconut. Run until mixture is smooth and scrape bowl as needed. Roll the mixture into 12 1-inch balls and roll in coconut to coat. Refrigerate at least 30 minutes.

Optional: You can roll Sinless Truffles in crushed almonds or walnuts in addition to or instead of coconut.

If you are using artificial sweeteners to lose weight, keep in mind that since the 1980s, consumption of artificial sweeteners and the rates of obesity have both soared considerably. Substituting a package of Sweet'n Low for a tablespoon of raw, unrefined sugar will not help you lose weight (one package of Sweet'n Low has 4 calories, whereas one teaspoon of sugar has 15 calories). Avoiding refined, processed goods that have added sugars such as high fructose corn syrup or sucrose and switching to a diet that consists of more natural sugars found in fruit and dairy products will facilitate weight loss. Although using sweeteners like Splenda occasionally is likely safe, it is best to turn to nature to get your sweet fix.

If you believe there is a link between the symptoms you are experiencing and an artificial sweetener such as aspartame, do not let others tell you it is all in your head. Simply follow a four–six–week elimination diet, where you remove the sweetener completely. Be sure to document the continuation or cessation of your symptoms.

Which is better — margarine or butter?

The debate of butter versus margarine has been going on for decades. Margarine first came on the scene in the early 1900s when food chemists discovered that heating refined vegetable oils in a process called *hydrogenation* and adding certain additives and coloring resulted in a spreadable and cheaper alternative to butter. Since then, many people have thought of margarine as a healthier option than butter. Healthcare practitioners often recommend using margarine because it is low in saturated fat and does not increase cholesterol. Unfortunately, this is the result of clever (or tricky!) marketing on behalf of the margarine companies. Margarine does indeed contain some saturated fat or it could not be hard at room temperature.

Margarine is created by transforming vegetable oils into unnatural forms that do not fit into the cellular membranes in our body. This change in shape, called the hydrogenation process, creates cellular damage throughout the body. Numerous research studies have found partially hydrogenated fats (or trans fatty acids) like margarine and shortening to increase the risk of arteriosclerosis, heart attack, cancer and stroke. Although margarine begins as a chemically extracted and refined vegetable oil, the final product contains manmade fats that promote inflammation throughout the body and raise the "bad cholesterol" known as LDL cholesterol.

Even though butter and margarine offer approximately the same amount of calories (35 calories and 4 grams of fat per teaspoon), my choice is always butter. In brief, butter is a more natural product whose chemical structure is very similar to the fats found in our body. Butter is an excellent source of fat-soluble vitamins such as vitamin A, D, E and K. People with a dairy sensitivity often tolerate butter quite well. This is due to the fact that butter is an almost pure fat and does not contain many of the allergens found in other milk products. Choose organic butter to avoid drug residue such as antibiotics being passed on from the cow. You will pay more money for butter than for margarine, but the health benefits (and taste it gives your food) is worth it!

You will find there is a teaspoon of butter used in some of our recipes here. Use butter sparingly as it is quite high in saturated fat (1 teaspoon is plenty to make your food taste delicious!). Also, consider using other oils, dips and spreads such as olive oil, hummus (chickpea spread) and low-fat or dairy-free cream cheese for your bread and cooking.

What about trans-fat-free margarine?

Certain margarine companies have developed trans-fat-free margarine. This means that each tablespoon of the spread contains no more than half a gram of trans fats. Although there is still a degree of trans fats in the product, it is certainly better than regular margarine. Typically, soft tub or liquid margarine is better than stick margarine. A tablespoon of stick margarine has about 1.9 grams of trans fat, while a tablespoon of regular tub margarine has approximately 0.8 grams of trans fats. Margarines that contain omega-3 and plant sterols to fight cholesterol are also available.

Is it healthy to drink alcohol? If so, what type and how much is recommended?

The research on alcohol's effect on health can be confusing. It appears that a small to moderate amount of alcohol daily may provide some benefits to health which include:

- Decrease in risk of heart disease or stroke
- Decrease in the development of peripheral vascular diseases
- Lowered risk of gallstones

What is a drink? A drink is defined as 12 ounces of beer, 5 ounces of wine or 1.5 ounces of distilled spirits. Anything more than a moderate amount of alcohol (i.e., 2 drinks per day) can have negative effects on health such as:

- Increased risk of breast or liver cancer
- Chronic pancreatitis
- Elevated triglyceride levels
- High blood pressure
- Cirrhosis of the liver
- Miscarriage
- Increased risk of suicide with excessive alcohol consumption
- Increased risk of injury or death due to motor vehicle accidents

For weight loss purposes, I am not an advocate of drinking daily (especially for women over the age of 40!). A daily drink can fluctuate blood sugars and tends to increase appetite. Trust me, I know that after a busy and hard day a glass of wine can certainly help to take the "edge off." However, daily alcohol consumption can quickly lead to an extra 5 to 10 pounds around our tummy area. I recommend limiting your alcoholic beverage intake to two to four drinks per week.

Are there additional health benefits to drinking red wine?

Red wine is a rich source of *phytochemicals* (plant chemicals) that have been shown to offer protection against various disease processes such as cancer and heart disease. The specific compounds found in red wine called *polyphenols,* such as *catechins* and *resveratrol* are thought to have significant antioxidant and anti-cancer properties. The French people's consumption of red wine is theorized to be one of the reasons their percentage of heart disease is so low (about one third less) in comparison to other countries such as the United States and Canada.

If you do not already consume alcohol, there is no reason you must start to reap the benefits. Pure purple grape juice (found in most health food stores) will also offer all the beneficial phytochemical effects.

I have heard eating chocolate can be good for your health. Is this true?

There are few foods that elicit as passionate a response as chocolate. True chocoholics crave a daily "fix" and feel an increase in mood and energy once the smallest amount of chocolate is eaten. This improvement in mood may be due to the fact that eating chocolate releases "feel good" chemicals called *endorphins.* Furthermore, chocolate stimulates the production of a brain chemical called *serotonin* which is a natural anti-depressant. Other health benefits of chocolate include:

- Essential trace elements and nutrients such as iron, calcium and potassium, and vitamins A, B1, C, D and E.
- One of the main ingredients of chocolate, cocoa, is also the highest natural source of magnesium. People who are magnesium deficient often report an intense chocolate craving.

In terms of chocolate, the darker, the better. Recent research has identified potent disease-fighting chemicals called *flavonoids* and *catechins* in the cocoa found in chocolate. These types of chemicals have been shown to be beneficial for heart health and in the prevention of free radical damage (damage to cells in the body) which can lead to various disease processes. In fact, dark chocolate (60 to 70 percent cocoa) contains twice the amount of antioxidants found in red wine and up to four times the amount found in green tea. Specifically, researchers found that dark chocolate contains 53.5 milligrams of catechins per 100 grams, whereas 100 milliliters of black tea contains a mere 13.9 milligrams of catechins.

Dark chocolate is slightly more expensive and is not as sweet as milk chocolate. However, milk chocolate and white chocolate contain more butterfat and fewer flavonoids in comparison to dark chocolate. For example:

- Dark chocolate = 53.5 milligrams of catechins per 100 grams
- White chocolate = 15.9 milligrams of catechins per 100 grams

It is also important to remember that although healthy, chocolate is high in saturated fat and is therefore high in calories. In addition, commercial chocolate bars are loaded with unwanted sugars, and "funny fats" such as trans fatty acids. I recommend purchasing a dark chocolate bar (60 to 70 percent cocoa) and freezing it in small squares. Grabbing a square or two per day will offer an abundant amount of disease-fighting chemicals and will satisfy even the most devoted chocoholic. You can also get your chocolate and fiber fix by eating two Dr. Joey Skinnychews per day.

How much fiber do I need to eat per day?

The amount of fiber recommended daily is between 25 and 30 grams. Two types of fiber are a necessary component of every diet. They are:

- **Soluble Fiber:** Includes oats and oat bran, dried beans and peas, fruits such as apples and oranges, vegetables such as carrots, and flaxseeds. Soluble fiber helps to regulate total cholesterol levels and LDL cholesterol (the "bad" cholesterol) in addition to controlling blood sugar levels (excellent for Type II diabetics).
- **Insoluble Fiber:** Includes wheat bran, 100 percent whole wheat products, flaxseeds, vegetables such as green beans and cauliflower, and fruit skins. Insoluble fiber is important for bowel health and to prevent or reverse constipation.

Foods containing at least 2 grams of fiber are considered a moderate source of fiber; at least 4 grams of fiber renders the food a high source and 6 grams or more of fiber per serving is a very high source of dietary fiber.

Do not concern yourself with getting different kinds of dietary fiber in varying amounts. Simply increasing your total fiber intake overall will be beneficial to your health. The following tips are helpful in boosting your fiber intake:

- Switch all of your grains to whole grain items.
- Sprinkle ground flaxseeds or bran cereal into a morning yogurt or shake daily.
- Eat a minimum of five to nine servings of fruits and veggies daily.
- Use beans in omelets, casseroles and salads, and eat bean dips such as hummus (chickpea spread). Green beans are especially high in fiber and are a great addition to casseroles or stir-fries.

Table 8.2: Grams of Fiber in Various Food Sources

Food	Fiber in Grams
1 medium apple	4
1 medium avocado	10
1 banana	3
1 cup of blackberries	7
1 medium orange	3
1/3 cup of All-Bran cereal	5.1
1 slice of whole grain bread	2
1/2 cup of baked beans	9.3
1/2 cup of lentils	3.7
1 tablespoon of flaxseed	2.5

I find it hard to eat breakfast in the morning. Is cereal or instant oatmeal a healthy way to start the day?

As mentioned previously, you *must* eat breakfast to lose weight and maintain proper blood sugar levels. Research clearly shows that breakfast skippers have difficulty losing weight. Even if you are not hungry, start your morning with a small meal.

People often find breakfast a tricky meal to eat healthfully. For this reason, I highly recommend getting into the habit of drinking a morning shake that contains all three macronutrients. For example, your morning shake could contain frozen or fresh fruit of your choice (low-glycemic carbohydrates), a scoop of protein powder, some almond milk or water and a teaspoon of flaxseed oil or ground flaxseeds (your essential fats). I even add a handful of spinach to my morning smoothie to get a "hit" of antioxidants. Morning shakes are quick and easy to prepare; they take a maximum of five minutes from start to finish (I prepare mine in under two minutes). One of my favorites is:

"LOOK 10 YEARS YOUNGER" SMOOTHIE (SERVES ONE)

This nutrient-dense detox smoothie will fill you up, optimize digestion and help you burn fat. The low-glycemic berries are filled to the brim with antioxidants and the ground flaxseeds offer fiber and omega-3. Enjoy!

- ½ cup unsweetened almond milk
- 4 tablespoons vanilla Greek yogurt
- ½ cup arugula or spinach
- 1 teaspoon green matcha powder
- ½ frozen banana

- ½ cup frozen berries
- 1 tablespoon ground flaxseeds

Mix all ingredients together. Blend on high for two minutes and enjoy!

Refer to the recipe section for more delicious and balanced breakfast ideas.

In addition to a morning power shake, there are other breakfast alternatives that will keep you energized and alert. However, a majority of quick breakfast options such as cereal and cereal bars are extremely carbohydrate dense, are made from refined flours and will fluctuate your blood sugar and insulin levels. By consuming them in the morning, you will feel tired and hungry early in the day; you may experience cravings and you will oversecrete insulin which leads to weight gain. Most cereals and cereal bars, with the exception of whole grain items (like All-Bran or slow-cooking oatmeal), are rated high on the Glycemic Index. Consider the following examples:

Table 8.3: The Glycemic Index for Breakfast Options

Low-Glycemic Breakfast Options	Moderate-Glycemic Breakfast Options	High-Glycemic Breakfast Options
Low-fat yogurt, 15	Mini Shredded Wheats, 58	Plain white baguette, 95
Grapefruit, 25	Bran Chex, 58	Cheerios, 74
Soymilk, 30	Bran muffin, 60	Cornflakes, 92
All-Bran, 30	Quick-cooking oatmeal, 65	Rice Krispies, 82
Oat Bran bread, 42	Instant oatmeal, 66	K-Time Just Right bar, 72
Old fashioned oatmeal, 49	Whole wheat bread, 69	

When eating a healthy breakfast, you still want to follow the Pick-3 System of eating which incorporates all three macronutrients: 1) low Glycemic Index carbohydrates, 2) lean proteins and 3) essential fats. In addition to the recipes outlined at the back of this book, balanced breakfast options include:

- Whole grain bread of choice with low-fat cream cheese spread or soy spread
- Low-fat yogurt with added fruit and walnuts
- Slow-cooking oatmeal with added protein powder, fruit and flax oil or ground flaxseeds
- Power shakes
- Omega-3 egg white omelet with whole grain bread (e.g., spelt bread)
- Omega-3 egg white omelet with vegetables
- Omega-3 poached egg on toast
- For a treat … omega-3 French toast (on whole grain bread) with maple syrup and yogurt on the side for protein

I get confused with serving sizes. What are common serving sizes for proteins, fats and carbohydrates?

Sample serving sizes of carbohydrates are:

- 1 serving of fruit (½ cup or 1 small fruit) = 10 grams of carbohydrates
- 1 cup of vegetables = 5 grams of carbohydrates
- ½ cup of beans = 20–25 grams of carbohydrates
- 1 whole wheat tortilla = 12 grams of carbohydrates

- 2 pieces of crisp Wasa bread = 15 grams of carbohydrates
- 1 slice of bread (whole wheat) = 15 grams of carbohydrates
- 1 bagel = 25–40 grams of carbohydrates depending on density

Sample serving sizes of protein are:

- 1 scoop of protein powder = 25 grams of protein
- 4 ounces of chicken or fish = 28 grams of protein
- 3 ounces of sirloin steak = 25 grams of protein
- ½ cup of egg whites = 13 grams of protein
- 1 ounce of low-fat cheese = 7 grams of protein
- 4 ounces of firm tofu = 10 grams of protein

Sample serving sizes of fats are:

- 1 teaspoon of extra virgin olive oil = 5 grams of fat
- 7 almonds = 5 grams of fat
- ⅛ of an avocado = 5 grams of fat
- 1 tablespoon of peanut butter = 5 grams of fat

What if I fall off the health wagon?

Whether it's during the weekend, a birthday party, a wedding or Christmas, we all fall off the health wagon and indulge in our favorite dessert, fried food or white fluffy croissant from time to time. When you do fall off the health wagon (not *if* you do; it happens to all of us!), do not beat yourself up with "food guilt." Do not think you have ruined all of the previous health advances that you had already made; you have not. Simply compensate the next day or the next meal by exercising balance. What do I mean by balance? Suppose you have eaten all the wrong foods until you are completely stuffed at a Thanksgiving meal. The next day jump back on the health wagon by:

- Starting your day with water and fresh-squeezed lemon to cleanse your system.
- Dropping all grains for two days, sticking to low-glycemic carbohydrates such as fruits and vegetables.
- Increasing your protein intake.
- Increasing your cardiovascular workout by 15 to 20 minutes.

How do I eat healthy if I am in a rush?

So many of us are in a rush these days—rushing to work, rushing the kids to soccer practice, rushing home to make dinner—you name it. We are zooming around like chickens with our heads cut off! When I see clients, I find they have a list of excuses as to why they cannot make nutritional changes. Topping the list is: "I don't have enough time." In fact, we are all busy people, but we need to make time for our health. Without it, nothing is as enjoyable as it should be.

Unless you dine out each and every meal, you have to grocery shop at least once a week. It does not take longer to pick healthy options over fast food or packaged products. I highly recommend grocery shopping on Sundays and getting your food ready for the week. I also recommend stocking your fridge and cupboards with "healthy grabables"—quick, easy and healthy snacks you can eat on the go. Although I am a strong advocate of sitting at a table and taking time to relax and enjoy the food you are about to eat, I realize this is not always realistic for people. Healthy grabables keep me eating healthily whether I am in the car, on an airplane or picking up my kids. They'll keep you eating healthily too.

HEALTHY GRABABLES

- Low-fat yogurt and nuts
- Protein bars—see Product Resource List
- Almonds
- Cashews
- Apples and cottage cheese
- Protein smoothie
- Sliced carrots and low-fat cheese
- Slices of low-fat cheese or goat cheese and walnuts
- Lean chicken breasts on multigrain bread with mustard
- All-Bran cereal and yogurt
- Cottage cheese and fruit
- Small containers of frozen vegetarian chili

How do I eat healthily when I am dining out?

When eating out, your caloric intake is increased. This is largely due to large portions, the use of oils and dressings you have no control over and our tendency to order and eat more when in a restaurant. In addition, to lure more customers, many restaurant establishments are "supersizing"—offering more food to appeal to consumers. Two-for-one slices of pizza, all-you-can-eat buffets and extra-large drinks are becoming the norm. In fact, research shows that the average restaurant meal is 765 calories while the average meal eaten at home is 425 calories. Compare some of the other statistics that highlight the downfalls of eating out:

- In 1996, 28 percent of young Americans said they had eaten out on any given day, compared to just 14 percent two decades earlier.
- The portion size of salty snacks has increased by 93 calories; soft drink size has grown by 49 calories and portions of French fries have swelled by 68 calories.

You can still eat healthily and follow the Pick-3 System of eating when dining out.

- Make sure to have a protein as part of your meal. Whether you choose salmon, lean beef, tofu, chicken or egg, protein will help keep your blood sugar levels in check.
- Skip the white bread and butter that is normally placed on the table at the beginning of the meal.
- Do not waste your carbohydrate grams or calories on juice or pop. Have bottled or bubbly water with lemon instead.
- Restaurants tend to go heavy on cheese and cheese sauces. If ordering a menu item that calls for cheese, ask your waiter to go light on the cheese. A healthier option to cheese sauce that is much lighter in fat and rich with lycopene (a cancer-fighting chemical) is a delicious, red tomato sauce.

- Include something fresh and "alive" in your meal like a tossed green salad or fruit plate.
- Stay away from cream-based soups loaded with trans fatty acids and saturated fat. Stick with soups that have a vegetable or chicken broth base or pureed soups.

With the surge in obesity and Type II diabetes, many fast food establishments are now offering healthier food options to the typical cheeseburger, fries and Coke menu—approximately 1340 calories or almost a day's worth of calories! While I do not think that fast-food restaurants should be a mainstay of anyone's diet, if you do occasionally eat fast food, being aware of healthier options available is important. See table 8.4 for suggestions.

Table 8.4: Healthy Alternatives

Instead of...	Try...
McDonald's medium French fries, 345 calories and 17 grams of fat	McDonald's side salad with Italian dressing, 72 calories and 4.1 grams of fat
McDonald's hot fudge sundae, 326 calories and 9.1 grams of fat	McDonald's fruit and yogurt parfait, 152 calories and 2.5 grams of fat
Burger King Original Whopper, 710 calories and 41 grams of fat	Burger King veggie burger, 300 calories and 7 grams of fat
Subway 6-inch cold cuts sub, 440 calories and 21 grams of fat	Subway 6-inch turkey breast sub (no cheese), 230 calories and 3 grams of fat

Why do I feel tired all day?

Fatigue is the "needle in a haystack" symptom that is somewhat tricky to get to the bottom of. In my years of practice, I have found that an individual's energy level, or lack of it, is intimately linked with the quality and quantity of their nutrition. I always tell people, "Eat alive to feel alive." A diet consisting of processed, fake and "dead" foods will make your energy plummet. Dragging yourself around all day and feeling unwell and sleepy on a regular basis is no way to live. Remember, unless there is an underlying medical issue, when given the right environment and conditions, the body will shift towards a state of health and wellness.

The four steps in this book are designed to get you to a state of energetic living. If you experience continual fatigue, explore your nutritional choices. Keep a food journal (refer to the appendix) in order to keep track of what and how much of a food you are eating. Although somewhat difficult to pinpoint, some common "energy zappers" are:

- A lack of water. Simply boosting your water in-take can often make energy levels soar.
- An abundant amount of high Glycemic Index foods in the diet. If you are slightly overweight, consider yourself insulin insensitive. If this is the case, eating highly refined high Glycemic Index foods will cause your blood sugar levels to bounce around and leave you feeling "crashed" throughout the day.
- A deficiency of protein. We do not crave protein. It is the comfort of carbohydrates found in breads, pastas, cookies or cakes that we crave. By adding a sufficient amount of protein to the diet you will help to balance your blood sugar levels and lose weight.
- A lack of exercise. You need to move to lubricate your joints, increase endorphin and energy

levels, and boost your metabolism.

- A lack of minerals and vitamins. Because most individuals do not eat enough fresh food, they lack certain minerals and vitamins. In addition, a large portion of the soil our produce is grown in has become tired and depleted. Thus, we do not receive the level of nutrition we once did.

- Lastly, drinking coffee leaches precious minerals and vitamins from the system. This is why I highly recommend investing in a high-quality multi-vitamin. See the Product Resource List for more information.

I have heard high-protein diets can be dangerous in the long term. Is this true?

There are pros and cons to high-protein diets. As we have seen, in order to increase metabolism and lose weight effectively, the Pick-3 System of eating outlined in chapter 4 is the most effective way to lose weight and keep it off. This system is not a high-protein diet; it is a moderate-protein diet. While it is higher in protein than recommended in Canada's Food Guide, which currently recommends five to 12 servings of grains and two to three servings of meat and alternatives, it is lower in protein than recommended in more extreme diets such Atkins or the Paleo diet.

The pros of high-protein diets are that you lose weight and boost metabolism quickly; however, it appears these diets are not sustainable for long periods of time and ultimately result in weight gain. Remember, each time you gain and lose weight your metabolism slows down, making future weight loss attempts harder and harder. It is far better to lose weight at a more gradual and sustained pace and keep it off permanently. I have been working with clients successfully in the weight loss world for over a decade. My two "pillars" when it comes to losing weight are:

1. Can you see yourself following a version of this program for the next five years? It does not make sense to keep jumping on and off programs. My hormonally-balanced weight loss approach (which incorporates the Pick-3 System of eating) is a shift that is made for life at any age.

2. You must lose weight with dignity! There are no injections or starvation diets, no weight loss bullying or feeling not good about yourself. Your weight loss journey is one that is personal and is a noble venture to undertake. Getting healthy and reclaiming your energy and vitality takes strength at first. The more support and information you can gather to help, the better. For more information, please visit www.shulmanweightloss.com.

The other downfall of high-protein diets is that the meals are often extremely high in red meat and fat. Overconsumption of red meat has been linked to osteoporosis, while overconsumption of saturated fat has been linked to heart disease, high blood pressure and an increase in cholesterol. Lastly, high-protein diets are often mineral-, vitamin- and fiber-deficient. It is not uncommon for an individual on a high-protein diet to experience constipation due to the lack of fiber.

The Pick-3 System of eating comprises:

- 40 percent low Glycemic Index carbohydrates (fruits, vegetables and whole grain items)
- 30 percent essential fats
- 30 percent lean proteins

Remember, if you have a question that has not been addressed, simply email me at www.drjoey.com.

appendix

Acid/Alkaline Foods

	ALKALIZING FOODS	
VEGETABLES	**FRUITS**	**OTHER**
Garlic	Apple	Apple Cider Vinegar
Asparagus	Apricot	Bee Pollen
Fermented Veggies	Avocado	Lecithin Granules
Watercress	Banana	Probiotic Cultures
Beets	Cantaloupe	Green Juices
Broccoli	Cherries	Veggie Juices
Brussels sprouts	Currants	Fresh Fruit Juice
Cabbage	Dates/Figs	Organic Milk (unpasteurized)
Carrot	Grapes	Mineral Water
Cauliflower	Grapefruit	Alkaline Antioxidant Water
Celery	Lime	Green Tea
Chard	Honeydew Melon	Herbal Tea
Collard Greens	Nectarine	Dandelion Tea
Cucumber	Orange	Ginseng Tea
Eggplant	Lemon	Banchi Tea
Kale	Peach	Kombucha
Kohlrabi	Pear	Chlorella
Lettuce	Pineapple	Spirulina
Mushrooms	Most Berries	
Mustard Greens	Tangerine	**SWEETENERS**
Dulce	Tomato	Stevia
Dandelions	Tropical Fruits	
Edible Flowers	Watermelon	**SPICES/SEASONINGS**
Onions		Cinnamon
Parsnips (high glycemic)	**PROTEIN**	Curry
Peas	Eggs	Ginger
Peppers	Whey Protein Powder	Mustard
Pumpkin	Cottage Cheese	Chili Pepper
Rutabaga	Chicken Breast	Sea Salt
Sea Veggies	Yogurt	Miso
Sprouts	Almonds	Tamari
Squashes	Chestnuts	All Herbs
Alfalfa	Tofu (fermented)	
Barley Grass	Flaxseeds	**ASIAN VEGETABLES**
Wheat Grass	Tempeh (fermented)	Maitake
Wild Greens	Squash Seeds	Daikon
Nightshade Veggies	Millet	Dandelion Root
	Sprouted Seeds	Shitake
	Nuts	Kombu
		Reishi
		Nori
		Umeboshi
		Wakame
		Sea Veggies

	ACIDIFYING FOODS	
FATS & OILS	**NUTS & BUTTERS**	**DRUGS & CHEMICALS**
Avocado Oil	Cashews	Drugs, Medicinal
Canola Oil	Brazil Nuts	Drugs, Psychedelic
Corn Oil	Peanuts	Chemicals, Pesticides
Flax Oil	Peanut Butter	Chemicals, Herbicides
Lard	Pecans	
Olive Oil	Tahini	**ALCOHOL**
Safflower Oil	Walnuts	Beer
Sesame Oil		Spirits
Sunflower Oil	**ANIMAL PROTEIN**	Wine
	Beef	
GRAINS	Carp	**BEANS & LEGUMES**
Rice Cakes	Clams	Black Beans
Wheat Cakes	Lamb	Chickpeas
Amaranth*	Lobster	Green Peas
Barley	Mussels	Kidney Beans
Buckwheat*	Oyster	Lentils
Corn*	Pork	Lima Beans
Oats (rolled)[1]*	Rabbit	Pinto Beans
Quinoa[2]*	Salmon	Red Beans
Rice (all)*	Shrimp	Soy Beans
Rye	Scallops	Soy Milk
Spelt	Tuna	White Beans
Kamut	Turkey	Rice Milk
Wheat	Venison	Almond Milk
Hemp Seed Flour		
Millet*	**FRUITS**	
Sorghum*	Cranberries	
Teff*		

*These grains are gluten-free.
[1]Make sure your oats are pure and uncontaminated.
[2]Quinoa is really a seed, although it looks and digests like a grain.

5-Day Food Diary

In order to accurately assess and monitor your dietary intake, it is critical to record what you have eaten on a daily basis. Use the following 5–Day Food Diary to record the amounts and types of food you eat, the water you drink and the supplements you take. You may also choose to record how you are feeling during the 5 days (i.e., energy, digestion, cravings, etc.) to reflect back on at a later date.

DAY 1

Breakfast

_____

_____

_____

_____

Lunch

_____

_____

_____

_____

Dinner

_____

_____

_____

_____

Snacks

_____

_____

_____

_____

# of glasses of water _____

Supplements taken (i.e., flaxseeds and acidophilus) _____

_____

_____

_____

Day 2

Breakfast

_____

_____

_____

_____

Lunch

_____

_____

_____

_____

Dinner

_____

_____

_____

_____

Snacks

_____

_____

_____

_____

# of glasses of water _____

Supplements taken (i.e., flaxseeds and acidophilus) _____

_____

_____

_____

DAY 3

Breakfast

_____

_____

_____

_____

Lunch

_____

_____

_____

_____

Dinner

_____

_____

_____

_____

Snacks

_____

_____

_____

_____

# of glasses of water _____

Supplements taken (i.e., flaxseeds and acidophilus) _____

_____

_____

_____

DAY 4

Breakfast

_____

_____

_____

_____

Lunch

_____

_____

_____

_____

Dinner

_____

_____

_____

_____

Snacks

_____

_____

_____

_____

# of glasses of water _____

Supplements taken (i.e., flaxseeds and acidophilus) _____

_____

_____

_____

DAY 5

Breakfast

_____

_____

_____

_____

Lunch

_____

_____

_____

_____

Dinner

_____

_____

_____

_____

Snacks

_____

_____

_____

_____

# of glasses of water _____

Supplements taken (i.e., flaxseeds and acidophilus) _____

_____

_____

_____

Glycemic Index and Glycemic Load

Value	Glycemic Index (GI)	Glycemic Load (GL)
High	70 or more	20
Medium	56 to 69 inclusive	11 to 19
Low	55 or less	10 or less

FRUITS AND FRUIT PRODUCTS:

Food Item	Glycemic Index (GI)	Glycemic Load (GL)
Apple	34	5
Apricots	57	5
Banana, ripe	51	13
Banana, under-ripe	30	6
Banana, over-ripe	48	12
Cantaloupe	65	4
Cherries	22	3
Cranberry juice	68	24
Dates, dried	103	42
Figs, dried	61	16
Grapefruit	25	3
Grapefruit juice, unsweetened	48	9
Grapes	46	8
Grapes, black	59	11
Kiwi fruit	53	6
Lychee, canned in syrup	79	16
Mango	51	8
Marmalade orange	48	9
Orange	42	5
Orange juice	52	12
Papaya	59	10
Peach	42	5

Peach, in heavy syrup	58	9
Pear	38	4
Pear halves, in syrup	25	4
Pineapple	59	7
Plum	39	5
Prunes, pitted	29	10
Raisins	64	28
Strawberries, fresh	40	1
Strawberry jam	51	10
Sultanas	56	25
Tomato juice, no sugar added	38	4
Watermelon	72	4

VEGETABLES:

Food Item	Glycemic Index (GI)	Glycemic Load (GL)
Broad beans	79	9
Green peas	48	3
Pumpkin	75	3
Sweet corn	54	9
Beet root	64	5
Carrots	71	3
Cassava, boiled	46	12
Parsnips	97	12
Baked potato	85	26
White potato, cooked	50	14
French fries, frozen	75	22
Instant mashed potato	85	17
New potato	57	12
Sweet potato	61	17

Note: The effect of vegetables such as broccoli, spinach and kale on blood sugar is negligible, and therefore they are not recorded in the GI or GL.

LEGUMES AND NUTS:

Food Item	Glycemic Index (GI)	Glycemic Load (GL)
Black-eye beans, boiled	42	13
Chick peas, boiled	28	8
Navy beans	38	12
Kidney beans, boiled	28	7
Black beans, cooked	20	5
Lentil, green boiled	30	5
Lentil, red, dried	26	5
Lima beans, frozen	32	10
Mung beans, cooked	42	7
Peas, dried, boiled	22	2
Pinto beans, dried	39	10
Romano beans	46	8
Soya beans, boiled	15	1
Split peas, boiled	32	6

BREADS:

Food Item	Glycemic Index (GI)	Glycemic Load (GL)
Bagel, white frozen	72	25
Baguette, white, plain	95	15
French baguette with chocolate spread	72	27
French baguette with butter and strawberry jam	62	26
Coarse barley kernel bread	27	5
Buckwheat bread	47	10
Hamburger bun	61	9
Kaiser roll	73	12
Gluten-free multigrain bread	79	10

Pumpernickel bread	46	5
Light rye	68	10
White spelt wheat bread	74	17
Spelt multigrain bread	54	7
White flour	70	10
100% whole grain bread	51	7

BREAKFAST CEREALS:

Food Item	Glycemic Index (GI)	Glycemic Load (GL)
All-Bran™	30	4
Bran Chex™	58	11
Cheerios™	74	15
Corn Bran™	75	15
Cornflakes™ (Kellogg's)	92	24
Corn Pop™ (Kellogg's)	80	21
Cream of Wheat™ (Nabisco)	66	17
Crispix™ (Kellogg's)	87	22
Froot Loops™ (Kellogg's)	69	18
Frosted Flakes™ (Kellogg's)	55	15
Grapenuts™ (Kraft)	67	13
Just Right™ (Kellogg's)	60	13
Mini Wheats™ (Kellogg's)	72	15
Muesli, No Name	60	11
Oat bran, raw	59	3
Porridge	69	16
Rice Krispies™ (Kellogg's)	82	21

recipes

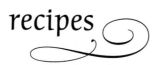

*I*n this section, you will find delicious recipe options for breakfast, lunch, dinner and snacks that are chock-full of nutrition. Considering the fact that most of us live busy, hectic lives, I realize it is not realistic to be cooking gourmet dishes in your kitchen. Because of this, you will find the recipes to be fast, delicious and easy to make. Designed by my husband (who is the best cook I know and is well known as "the shortcut chef"), most of the recipes you will find take under 30 minutes to prepare—some can even be made in under five minutes! Of course, you can switch a meal option and eat it at any time of day. So … if you feel like having eggs for dinner or salmon for lunch—go for it!

There are a few tricks of the trade that will help you permanently fit healthy eating into your life. I assure you, once you start feeling well and energetic and looking your very best, you will only want to continue climbing the ladder of health. The following suggestions will work to keep your diet on track, with inner health and outer beauty as the long-lasting results.

- Bring healthy snacks to work that are easy to "grab." These include nuts, seeds, healthy bars, cut-up fruits, vegetables and "to go" soups.
- Organize a food list and grocery shop a minimum of once per week. This will ensure your home is stocked with healthy and fresh food items.
- Visit the bulk section of your grocery store and load up on healthy goodies such as chopped walnuts, sliced almonds (they're delicious toasted!), trail mix, soy nuts and seeds that can be

sprinkled over a salad. Most bulk sections also have whole grain flour or pasta such as spelt or kamut and organic soup mixes.

- Cut up vegetables such as celery, broccoli florets, cauliflower and carrots and keep them in your fridge. When you are craving a munchie, grab a veggie.
- Do not be afraid to spice it up! Using spices is one of the best methods to flavor your food.

Please Note:

- All recipes outlined below serve two.
- The nutrition facts given for each recipe are for one individual serving only (i.e., amount of calories, fat, carbohydrate and protein grams eaten per person).
- Certain recipes are not suitable to eat during the five-day cleanse due to their grain or dairy content. Please refer to the end of chapter 3 for meal options during your cleansing period.
- (☺) = Dish can be eaten during the five-day cleanse.

Breakfast

TRIPLE BERRY SHAKE (☺)

Minutes to Prepare: 5

Ingredients
½ cup frozen mixed berries
½ small frozen banana
¼ cup almond or rice milk, unsweetened
2 scoops protein powder
2 teaspoons flaxseed oil
2 handfuls of spinach

Directions
Combine all ingredients and blend on high for 90 seconds.

Nutritional Facts Per Serving
Total calories: 250
Protein: 20 grams
Carbohydrates: 25 grams
Fat: 6 grams

Recipe Tip: Researchers at the USDA Human Nutrition Research Center on Aging (HNRCA) have found that blueberries rank #1 in antioxidant activity when compared to 40 other fresh fruits and vegetables. Antioxidants help to neutralize harmful by-products called free radicals that can lead to cancer and other age-related diseases.

COFFEE BANANA MORNING SMOOTHIE

Minutes to Prepare: under 5

Ingredients

1 frozen banana

1½ cups fat-free milk or unsweetened almond milk

4 ounces low-fat coffee yogurt

¼ teaspoon cinnamon

2 scoops protein powder

2 teaspoons ground flaxseeds

Directions

Combine all ingredients and blend on high for 90 seconds.

Nutritional Facts Per Serving

Total calories: 285

Protein: 25 grams

Carbohydrates: 27 grams

Fat: 6 grams

Recipe Tip: Take apart your blender and wash it thoroughly once per week. By doing so, you will avoid the risk of bacterial build-up.

CREAMY VANILLA PROTEIN DELIGHT (☺)

Minutes to Prepare: under 5

Ingredients
1 cup almond milk, unsweetened
4 ounces coconut yogurt
1 small frozen banana
2 teaspoons pure vanilla extract
2 scoops French vanilla whey protein powder
2 teaspoons flaxseed oil or ground flaxseeds
cinnamon to taste

Directions
Combine all ingredients and blend on high for 90 seconds.

Nutritional Facts Per Serving
Total calories: 300
Protein: 23 grams
Carbohydrates: 27 grams
Fat: 9 grams

Recipe Tip: Vanilla or chocolate protein powder is an excellent option to get your "sweet fix" without raising insulin or blood sugar levels. Remember, an oversecretion of insulin results in excess fat and fatigue. Refer to the Product Resource List for protein powder recommendations.

WHOLE GRAIN BREAD, LOX AND CREAM CHEESE

Minutes to Prepare: 5

Note: This recipe serves one.

Ingredients
2 slices sprouted-grain bread
2 teaspoons light cream cheese
3 ounces wild smoked salmon
sliced red tomatoes and cucumbers
1 tablespoon capers

Directions
Spread cream cheese on bread. Add lox, sliced tomatoes, cucumbers and capers on top.

Nutritional Facts Per Serving
Total calories: 262
Protein: 24 grams
Carbohydrates: 26 grams
Fat: 6 grams

Recipe Tip: Large-scale studies have shown farmed salmon to contain excessive levels of organic pollutants called PCBs. In order to reap the benefits from eating salmon which offers omega-3 fats and an excellent source of lean protein, I recommend splurging on wild salmon. Not only is the toxic load of the fish significantly less, the taste is noticeably fresher and smoother.

POWER BANANA OATMEAL

Minutes to Prepare: 15

Ingredients

⅔ cup slow-cooking oats

1½ cups water

2 20-gram scoops vanilla-flavored
      protein powder

1 medium-sized ripe banana

1 tablespoon natural brown sugar

1 cup almond or rice milk,
   unsweetened

2 teaspoons ground flaxseeds

Directions

Pour water into the saucepan and place on high heat to boil. Add slow-cooking oats and stir. Bring the mixture to a boil again, then reduce heat and simmer for 10 to 15 minutes. Remove from heat. Peel banana and slice thinly. Add to cooked oatmeal. Add protein powder and mix thoroughly. Divide mixture between two bowls, sprinkle brown sugar and flaxseeds over top and add ½ cup of almond or rice milk to each bowl. Serve and eat.

Nutritional Facts Per Serving

Total calories: 300

Protein: 22 grams

Carbohydrates: 40 grams

Fat: 5 grams

Recipe Tip: Slow-cooking oats are chock-full of nutrition, offering high amounts of B vitamins, calcium, protein and fiber while being low in salt and unsaturated fat. Due to their rich fiber content, slow-cooking oats also rank lower on the Glycemic Index in comparison to instant oatmeal. A morning meal of slow-cooking oats with added protein powder will not zap your energy the way instant oatmeal does and will not cause you to gain weight.

APPLES AND CINNAMON PROTEIN OATMEAL

Minutes to Prepare: 15

Ingredients

⅔ cup slow-cooking oats

1½ cups water

2 20-gram scoops protein powder

2 medium apples, peeled, cored and diced

2 teaspoons cinnamon

1 tablespoon natural cane sugar

1 cup almond milk, unsweetened

2 teaspoons ground flaxseeds

Directions

Pour water into saucepan and place on high heat. Bring water to boil. Add slow-cooking oats and stir. Bring mixture to a boil again, then reduce heat and simmer for 10 to 15 minutes. Remove from heat. Peel and core apples. Cut into small cubes and add to cooking oatmeal after 5 minutes. Also add protein powder and mix thoroughly. Divide mixture between two bowls, sprinkle cinnamon and cane sugar over top and add ½ cup of almond milk to each bowl. Serve and eat.

Nutritional Facts Per Serving

Total calories: 300

Protein: 22 grams

Carbohydrates: 40 grams

Fat: 5 grams

Recipe Tip: In a hurry? One trick is to prepare five days' worth of oatmeal in advance. Store in an airtight container in your refrigerator and use as required. To reheat, use a microwave; heat on high for two to three minutes and enjoy!

GOOD MORNING FRUIT AND COTTAGE CHEESE

Minutes to Prepare: 5

Ingredients

1½ cups 1% cottage cheese

¼ cup sliced fresh strawberries

¼ cup fresh blueberries

1 medium banana, sliced

4 teaspoons Bran Buds

4 teaspoons sliced almonds

Directions

Divide cottage cheese into two bowls. Wash strawberries, remove stems and slice thinly. Wash blueberries and slice banana. Divide fruit evenly into cottage cheese and stir. Sprinkle Bran Buds and sliced almonds over top and serve.

Nutritional Facts Per Serving

Total calories: 250

Protein: 23 grams

Carbohydrates: 27 grams

Fat: 5 grams

Recipe Tip: Low-fat or 1% cottage cheese offers an excellent source of protein, is low in calories and high in bone-building calcium. Cottage cheese should be used promptly and will only stay fresh for one week maximum in the fridge.

BROCCOLI CHEESY EGGS (☺) (Omit bread and use goat cheese for five–day cleanse.)

Minutes to Prepare: 15

Ingredients

1 medium egg

1 cup egg whites

½ white onion

1½ cups broccoli florets

1 teaspoon butter

2 ounces plain goat cheese

2 slices whole grain bread, toasted

¼ teaspoon salt

¼ teaspoon pepper

Directions

Crack egg into a medium–sized mixing bowl. Add egg whites and mix thoroughly with a whisk. Peel and dice onion. Remove stems from broccoli and cut florets into small pieces. Melt butter in a non-stick pan on medium–high heat. Add diced onion and broccoli. Continue stirring until broccoli begins to become tender but is still a bit crunchy. Pour egg mixture on top of onions and broccoli. Stir constantly. When the egg mixture is half cooked, add salt and pepper and goat cheese. Continue to cook until the egg mixture is fully cooked. Garnish with tomato slices and enjoy with one slice of toasted whole grain bread each.

Nutritional Facts Per Serving

Total calories: 230

Protein: 25 grams

Carbohydrates: 18 grams

Fat: 7.5 grams

Recipe Tip: Onions have been used for their medicinal properties for centuries. They have antibacterial and antifungal properties, and a paste or an ointment made out of onion is said to prevent infection in wounds and burns. For health benefits and a wonderful flavor, try to include onions and garlic in as many recipes as you can.

TEX-MEX EGGS (☺) (Omit bread for the five-day cleanse.)

Minutes to Prepare: 15

Ingredients

3 omega-3 eggs	3 slices veggie salami, diced
½ cup egg whites	Tex-Mex seasoning
½ cup chopped broccoli	1 teaspoon butter
1 medium onion, diced	2 slices whole grain bread

Directions

In a medium-sized frying pan, sauté onion, broccoli, butter and veggie salami until tender. Mix the egg, egg whites and Tex-Mex seasoning together and add to the frying pan. Cook on medium-high heat. Stir constantly until cooked and serve with a slice of toasted whole grain bread on the side (lightly buttered if desired).

Nutritional Facts Per Serving
Total calories: 300
Protein: 31 grams
Carbohydrates: 21 grams
Fat: 9 grams

> **Recipe Tip:** Vegetarian meat products are now available as hamburgers, hot dogs, pepperoni and salami! High in protein and low in saturated fat and calories, soy-based "meats" do not cause clogging of the arteries or inflammation. As an occasional option, they can be included in the diet.

WHOLE GRAIN OMEGA-3 FRENCH TOAST

Minutes to Prepare: 10

Ingredients

4 slices of whole grain bread

2 omega-3 eggs

½ cup egg whites

1 teaspoon butter

1 teaspoon cinnamon

6 teaspoons natural maple syrup

½ cup sliced strawberries

Directions

Crack eggs and egg whites into a medium-sized bowl and beat with a whisk until completely blended. Add cinnamon and continue to beat. Place a small amount of butter into a non-stick frying pan and melt. One at a time, dip whole grain bread into the egg mixture. Allow each bread slice to soak for 20 to 30 seconds in the egg mixture. Flip them over and repeat the process. Then carefully remove each piece of egg-soaked bread from the bowl and place in the preheated frying pan on medium-high heat. Allow to cook for approximately two minutes on each side. Place on a serving plate. Top with sliced strawberries, drizzle with maple syrup and serve.

Nutritional Facts Per Serving

Total calories: 270

Protein: 17 grams

Carbohydrates: 38 grams

Fat: 7 grams

> **Recipe Tip:** Made with whole grains and omega-3 eggs, this recipe is a much healthier version of French toast. However, it is slightly higher in carbohydrates in comparison to other recipes and should be eaten as a weekend treat instead of as an everyday meal.

Lunch

WHOLE GRAIN TURKEY AVOCADO SANDWICH

Note: This recipe serves one.

Minutes to Prepare: 5

Ingredients

2 slices whole grain bread

¼ avocado, sliced

4 slices of fresh roasted turkey

4 slices each of tomato and cucumber

1 teaspoon Dijon mustard

salt and pepper to taste

4 ounces low-fat yogurt

Directions

Toast bread and spread on Dijon mustard. Serve open face, placing turkey, avocado, tomato and cucumber slices on bread. Add salt and pepper to taste. Enjoy with a low-fat yogurt for dessert!

Nutritional Facts Per Serving

Total calories: 400

Protein: 33 grams

Carbohydrates: 42 grams

Fat: 11 grams

> **Recipe Tip:** Avocados are chock-full of the "good fat" monounsaturated fat, which has been shown to lower the bad cholesterol (LDL) and boost the good cholesterol (HDL). They are a wonderful alternative to spread on a piece of whole grain bread or to eat in slices in salads or sandwiches. Avocados can also be used to make guacamole—a delicious dip for vegetables and baked nachos. To ripen an avocado, simply place it in a paper bag with a banana or apple at room temperature until ready to eat in about two to five days.

TUNA WRAPS

Minutes to Prepare: 5

Ingredients

4 small whole grain wraps

1 can drained light tuna

½ cup chopped romaine lettuce

¼ diced white onion

½ large ripe tomato

1 tablespoon light mayonnaise

salt and pepper to taste

½ teaspoon cumin

1 small container of yogurt

Directions

Mix drained tuna, salt, pepper, cumin and light mayonnaise in a deep container and blend thoroughly with a hand blender. Spoon mixture, distributed evenly, down the center of the four wraps. Cover with onion, tomato and romaine lettuce, wrap and serve. Enjoy with a serving of yogurt on the side.

Nutritional Facts Per Serving (2 wraps)

Total calories: 373

Protein: 27 grams

Carbohydrates: 43 grams

Fat: 10 grams

Recipe Tip: When purchasing tuna, select *light* albacore tuna instead of *white* tuna which has been shown to be higher in mercury content. An excess of mercury has been linked to neurological disorders, autism and learning delays in children. According to the FDA, pregnant women, nursing mothers and young children should limit themselves to 12 ounces of fish per week (2 regular servings) from fish sources which are lower in mercury content. These include shrimp, canned light tuna, salmon, pollock and catfish.

SALMON CAESAR SALAD

Minutes to Prepare: 20

Ingredients

2 4-ounce salmon fillets

4 pieces of whole grain toast

1 large head of romaine lettuce

3 tablespoons of Caesar
   dressing (page 77)

garlic powder

2 teaspoons Parmesan cheese

½ teaspoon of butter

salt and pepper to taste

1 fresh lemon

dillseed to taste

Directions

Break romaine lettuce into coarse pieces. Butter whole grain toast and sprinkle with garlic powder. Bake in at 375 degrees F until golden brown. Let bread cool and cut into small pieces for croutons.

Grease baking sheet and place salmon on it. Sprinkle salmon with salt and pepper and squeeze ½ lemon over both fillets. Sprinkle dillseed on salmon with ¼ teaspoon of butter on each fillet. Cover with 2 thin slices of fresh lemon. Broil in oven for 20 minutes.

Slice up salmon and combine lettuce, croutons, salmon, dressing and Parmesan cheese. Serve and enjoy.

Nutritional Facts Per Serving

Total calories: 310

Protein: 30 grams

Carbohydrates: 28 grams

Fat: 10 grams

Recipe Tip: Nobody likes their salmon to taste "fishy." In order to ensure you get the best taste from your fillet, remove the skin prior to broiling.

CHUNKY CHICKEN SALAD (☺)

Minutes to Prepare: 40

Ingredients

2 boneless chicken breasts

1 cup diced celery

1 cup diced apple

¼ cup sultana raisins

¼ finely diced red onion

¼ cup chopped walnuts

2 tablespoons light mayonnaise

¼ teaspoon salt

¼ teaspoon pepper

½ teaspoon sage

Directions

Coat chicken breasts with salt, pepper and sage. Bake or barbeque chicken breasts until done. Chill and cut into cubes. Peel and dice apple, dice celery and finely chop red onion and walnuts. Combine all ingredients, including raisins and mayonnaise. Stir until evenly mixed, chill and serve.

Nutritional Facts Per Serving

Total calories: 400

Protein: 27 grams

Carbohydrates: 32 grams

Fat: 14 grams

Recipe Tip: Although fat contains more than two times the amount of calories in comparison to carbohydrates and protein (9 calories versus the 4 calories found in carbohydrates and protein), certain fats such as omega-3 essential fats are extremely beneficial to your health. In fact, a cup of walnuts provides 90.8 percent of the daily value for omega-3 essential fat. Walnuts also contain an antioxidant compound called *ellagic acid* that supports the immune system and appears to have several anti-cancer properties.

Salmon-Mango Wraps

Minutes to Prepare: 15

Ingredients

4 small whole grain wraps

1 can wild Atlantic salmon, drained

½ cup chopped romaine lettuce

¼ diced white onion

1 whole mango, peeled and chopped

½ fresh red pepper, chopped

½ large ripe tomato

1 tablespoon mango dressing
    (page 248)

salt and pepper to taste

Directions

Break salmon into small chunks with a fork and remove bones. (This is by preference only—the bones actually provide a good source of calcium.) Add mango pieces and mango dressing and mix thoroughly. Spoon mixture down the center of the four whole grain wraps. Top with lettuce, onion, tomato and red pepper. Add salt and pepper to taste. Fold wraps and serve.

Nutritional Facts Per Serving (2 small wraps)

Total calories: 420

Protein: 27 grams

Carbohydrates: 48 grams

Fat: 12 grams

Recipe Tip: Whole grain foods contain nutrients to increase immune system function and boost energy such as vitamins B and E, iron and magnesium. In addition, whole grain foods have been found to help lower cholesterol and are beneficial for weight loss. To identify products that are whole grain, check the ingredients list for the words "whole" or "whole grain" before the name of the grain, for instance, "whole wheat" or "whole grain oats."

Chicken Caesar Sandwich

Minutes to Prepare: 10

Ingredients

4 slices of multigrain bread

6 ounces cooked sliced chicken breast

2 slices low-fat or veggie cheese slices

4 slices tomato

½ avocado

½ cup thinly shredded romaine lettuce

2 teaspoons Caesar dressing (page 77)

salt and pepper to taste

Directions

Toast multigrain bread. Heat chicken slices in non-stick pan or in microwave.

Mash avocado, divide evenly and spread on each slice of bread. Coat bread with Caesar dressing and top with tomato slices, shredded lettuce, and salt and pepper to taste. Divide cooked sliced chicken and place on bread. Cut sandwiches in half and serve with cucumber slices.

Nutritional Facts Per Serving

Total calories: 370

Protein: 28 grams

Carbohydrates: 31 grams

Fat: 14 grams

Recipe Tip: *Lycopene* is a chemical responsible for tomatoes' rich red color. Lycopene has also been strongly linked to a reduced risk of prostate, rectal and colon cancer. This disease-fighting chemical is best absorbed in the presence of fat, so adding a small amount of olive oil to your tomato or tomato-based products will strengthen lycopene's powerful effects.

TEMPTING TEMPEH SALAD (☺)

Minutes to Prepare: 15

Ingredients
Salad

500-gram package of tempeh

3 cups romaine lettuce, washed and broken into 2-inch pieces

1 medium apple, peeled, cored and diced

1 mango, peeled and diced

¼ seedless cucumber, diced

¼ cup walnuts

¼ cup fresh cilantro, finely chopped

1 cup cherry tomatoes

Dressing

1 mango, peeled and diced

4 tablespoons extra virgin olive oil

3 tablespoons chopped white onion

salt and pepper to taste

Directions
Salad: Cut tempeh into cubes. Mix romaine lettuce, mango pieces, apple, cucumber, walnuts, cherry tomatoes and tempeh in a bowl and toss. Pour dressing over salad just before serving.

Dressing: Mix diced mango, onion, olive oil and salt and pepper in a food processor. If you do not have a food processor, a hand blender will work just as well. Blend until creamy.

Nutritional Facts Per Serving (including dressing)
Total calories: 362
Protein: 18 grams
Carbohydrates: 46 grams
Fat: 15 grams

Recipe Tip: Tempeh has been a food staple in Indonesia for over 2,000 years. It is made from fermented soybeans mixed with grains, usually rice or millet, and then incubated with a starter to begin the fermentation process. Tempeh is a wonderful substitute for meat as it is very high in protein and low in fat and carbohydrates. Its firm texture and nutty taste make it perfect to grill or barbeque, add to stir-fries or use instead of a beef patty.

Mexicasa Egg Wraps

Minutes to Prepare: 15

Ingredients

2 whole eggs

6 egg whites

4 whole grain or high-protein wraps

¼ head romaine lettuce

1 ripe tomato

1 tablespoon Tex-Mex seasoning

4 tablespoons salsa

1 teaspoon butter

Directions

Break whole eggs into a mixing bowl. Combine with egg whites and Tex-Mex seasoning and blend with a whisk. Melt butter into non-stick pan and add egg mixture. Cook on medium-high heat. Continue to stir until mixture is cooked. Brown wraps on both sides in a clean pan over medium-high heat. Shred lettuce with a chopping knife. Dice tomatoes. Spread out wraps and distribute the egg mixture evenly. Spoon salsa evenly over egg mixture. Top with chopped lettuce and tomato. Fold the wraps and serve.

Nutritional Facts Per Serving (2 wraps)

Total calories: 360

Protein: 25 grams

Carbohydrates: 36 grams

Fat: 12 grams

Recipe Tip: Salsa is a wonderful low-glycemic condiment to use on meats, vegetables and eggs. This low-calorie condiment contains only 2 calories per teaspoon!

Tasty Tuna and Pasta Salad

Minutes to Prepare: 15

Ingredients

1 can tuna (120 grams or 4 ½ ounces)   ½ diced red pepper

½ cup diced white onion   ½ avocado

8 ounces kamut pasta (rotini)   ¼ teaspoon garlic

2 tablespoons light mayonnaise   salt and pepper to taste

½ cup diced celery

Directions

Add pasta to 2 quarts of boiling water and cook for 9 to 12 minutes or per package instructions. Remove from heat and cool in running cold water. Combine tuna, onion, mayonnaise, diced celery, red pepper, garlic, salt and pepper in a mixing bowl. Mix thoroughly and refrigerate. Slice the avocado in half, remove the pit, then peel and slice into 1-inch slices. Spoon the tuna salad mixture onto a plate. Top with avocado slices and serve.

Nutritional Facts Per Serving (2 wraps)

Total calories: 429

Protein: 30 grams

Carbohydrates: 40 grams

Fat: 10 grams

Recipe Tip: Mayonnaise is of French origin and is made of oil, egg yolks, vinegar and seasoning. It contains 0 grams of trans fats and is a source of omega-3 and vitamin E.

HEALTHY PIZZA BAKE

Minutes to Prepare: 10

Ingredients

4 slices whole grain bread

4 slices soy or low-fat cheese

½ cup chopped white mushrooms

½ chopped white onion

1 tablespoon olive oil

1 teaspoon chopped garlic

4 tablespoons spaghetti sauce or
   pizza sauce

salt and pepper to taste

dried oregano

Directions

Toast multigrain bread in a toaster. Sauté the garlic, onion and mushrooms in olive oil until golden brown. Coat each piece of bread with spaghetti or pizza sauce. Evenly distribute onion/mushroom mixture on top. Sprinkle with oregano, salt and pepper. Place a slice of soy or low-fat cheese on top. Bake in a preheated oven at 415 degrees until cheese melts. Combine with a flavored yogurt for dessert!

Nutritional Facts Per Serving (2 pieces of whole grain bread)

Total calories: 300

Protein: 25 grams

Carbohydrates: 40 grams

Fat: 7 grams

Recipe Tip: Go for garlic! Garlic has a long history of being a powerful natural antibiotic and is beneficial to the cardiovascular system. The medicinal properties and benefits of garlic are strongest when eaten raw—crushed or very finely chopped. But don't overdo it; garlic can be hard on the digestive system.

Dinner

SWEET POTATO SALMON CAKES

Minutes to Prepare: 35

Ingredients

8 ounces red salmon, preferably wild Atlantic salmon

2 medium sweet potatoes, peeled and steamed

1 medium onion, peeled and diced

½ teaspoon dillseed

1 tablespoon butter

1 egg

¼ cup breadcrumbs

salt and pepper to taste

Directions

Peel and cube sweet potatoes. Steam for 30 minutes and allow to cool. While the sweet potatoes are cooling, peel and dice onion; then sauté it in 1 teaspoon of butter. Combine salmon, sweet potato, breadcrumbs, egg, salt, pepper, dillseed and sautéed onions in a bowl and blend with a potato masher.

Melt the balance of the butter in a non-stick frying pan. Form salmon into flat patties, approximately 3 inches in diameter. Dust with breadcrumbs and cook in a non-stick pan until golden brown. Serve immediately.

Nutritional Facts Per Serving

Total calories: 420
Protein: 30 grams
Carbohydrates: 45 grams
Fat: 12 grams

> **Recipe Tip:** As a general rule, the more colorful the fruit or vegetable, the healthier it is. Chemicals (called phytochemicals) give fruits and vegetables their vibrant hues of green, orange, red and purple and are responsible for disease-fighting properties. Sweet potatoes are loaded with beta carotene, vitamin E, vitamin B6, potassium and iron.

MANGO CHUTNEY CHICKEN

Minutes to Prepare: 25

Ingredients

2 boneless/skinless chicken breasts

1 large ripe mango

1 large ripe tomato

¼ red onion

1 tablespoon olive oil

1 tablespoon cane sugar

4 tablespoons fresh cilantro

1 teaspoon butter

½ teaspoon poultry seasoning

1 teaspoon finely minced jalapeño
  pepper—if desired (spicy hot)

salt and pepper to taste

Directions

Mango Chutney: Peel and dice mango into ½-inch cubes. Cube and dice tomato into ½-inch cubes. Finely dice red onion and cilantro. Add olive oil, jalapeño pepper, salt and pepper and mix thoroughly. With a hand blender, puree one-quarter of the mixture and set aside.

Chicken: Melt butter and coat chicken breasts. Sprinkle chicken liberally with poultry seasoning, salt and pepper. Wrap the chicken in aluminum foil and place on the barbeque* on high heat for 8 minutes. The chicken will cook completely through and seal the juices in. Open up the aluminum foil and spoon on the pureed mango chutney. Continue to barbeque on medium-high for 8 more minutes. When the chicken is done, place it on a plate and cover with the balance of the mango chutney and serve. Enjoy with a side salad.

*You can substitute your oven for the barbeque. Set at 425 degrees.

Recipe Tip: The Mediterranean diet is considered to be one of the healthiest diets in the world. It consists of a large amount of fruits, vegetables, beans, whole grains and a low to moderate amount of chicken, fish, dairy and even red wine! Another aspect of the Mediterranean diet that has been shown to have cholesterol-lowering and heart-healthy effects is the inclusion of the monounsaturated fat olive oil.

Nutritional Facts Per Serving

Total calories: 355

Protein: 26 grams

Carbohydrates: 39 grams

Fat: 11 grams

Recipe Tip: When choosing olive oil, be sure to pick extra virgin olive oil. This is from the first pressing of the olive. In general, the darker the oil, the more flavorful. Light olive oils are best used for high-heat frying, whereas regular olive oil is better suited for low- to medium-heat cooking as well as for many uncooked foods such as salad dressings and marinades.

PORTOBELLO TUNA MELT

Minutes to Prepare: 20

Ingredients

2 cans light flaked tuna, drained and set aside

4 Portobello mushrooms, center stem removed

1 medium cooking onion

½ cup white sliced mushrooms

1 teaspoon minced garlic

1 teaspoon butter

4 slices soy or low-fat cheese

salt and pepper to taste

4 pieces whole grain bread

Note: If you want to spice up your meal, add ¼ teaspoon of cayenne pepper.

Directions

Chop onions and mushrooms and sauté in butter with garlic. Mix with tuna; add salt and pepper to taste (use cayenne pepper if desired). Spoon equal portions of the tuna mixture on each mushroom cap. Bake for 20 minutes at 400 degrees. Place a cheese slice on top of each mushroom. Bake for 3 or 4 more minutes and serve with toasted whole grain bread on the side.

Nutritional Facts Per Serving (2 pieces of bread each)

Total calories: 470

Protein: 53 grams

Carbohydrates: 36 grams

Fat: 14 grams

Recipe Tip: Portobello mushrooms offer a great alternative to bread. With their "meaty taste" they are filling and are a good source of protein and an excellent source of niacin (vitamin B3). Use Portobello mushrooms promptly, or store them in a brown paper bag in your fridge. They will keep for 7 to 10 days.

Egg Drop Soup

Minutes to Prepare: 20

Ingredients

1 liter box organic chicken broth

2 cups water

1 medium onion, diced

1 cup sliced mushrooms

1 medium broccoli, florets only

4 medium carrots, sliced

2 large stalks of celery diced

3 omega-3 eggs

1 cup extra firm low-fat tofu

1 tablespoon butter

salt and pepper to taste

Directions

Chop all vegetables and cut extra firm tofu into small cubes. Mix water and chicken broth. Combine all ingredients except the eggs. Cook on high heat until the broth begins to boil. Reduce to medium heat for 8 to 10 minutes, until the vegetables are tender. Crack eggs one at a time and pour into the soup mixture. Try to ensure the yolks are broken before dropping eggs into the soup. Gently stir soup to ensure the egg is evenly distributed and cooked. Add more salt and pepper to taste.

Note: Because extra water is added to the soup base, a fair bit of salt is required to achieve the right taste.

Nutritional Facts Per Serving

Total calories: 423

Protein: 34 grams

Carbohydrates: 38 grams

Fat: 10 grams

Recipe Tip: When shopping for eggs, make sure to purchase omega-3 eggs which offer 300 to 400 mg of the essential fat omega-3! In addition to making your complexion more radiant and your hair softer, omega-3 fats have been shown to be beneficial for allergies, attention deficit disorder, depression, weight loss and heart disease. They can even boost your immune system function.

DILL SALMON BAKE WITH CREAMY CAULIFLOWER

Minutes to Prepare: 40

Ingredients

Salmon

2 4-ounce boneless and skinless   1 fresh lemon
   salmon fillets   salt and pepper
2 large sprigs dill

Creamy Cauliflower

½ head cauliflower   1 whole onion, chopped
½ cup skim milk   1 cup fresh chopped mushrooms
1 tablespoon + 1 teaspoon butter   1 teaspoon minced garlic
½ teaspoon onion powder   3 tablespoons whole wheat flour
1 cup grated soy or low-fat cheese

Directions

Salmon: Grease baking sheet. Squeeze juice from ½ lemon over salmon fillets. Sprinkle on salt and pepper. Place 2 sprigs of dill on the fillets and top with 2 thin slices of lemon. Place under the broiler for 15 to 20 minutes. Place fillets on plate (garnish with lettuce and tomato if desired).

Creamy Cauliflower: Cut cauliflower into florets and place in steamer for 30 minutes. In a separate pot combine milk, 1 tablespoon butter, onion powder and cheese, and place over medium–high heat. Whisk the sauce continually to avoid burning. Bring to a boil and continue to whisk until the cheese is melted. In a separate cup, add flour to 6 ounces of water. Whisk until smooth. Begin pouring flour mixture into the boiling cheese mix until desired consistency is achieved.

Pan fry mushrooms and onions with 1 teaspoon of butter and add garlic, salt and pepper. Coarsely chop the steamed cauliflower. Top with the onion and mushroom mixture and drizzle cheese sauce over it all and serve. Enjoy with a slice of whole wheat bread.

Nutritional Facts Per Serving
Total calories: 355
Protein: 26 grams
Carbohydrates: 39 grams
Fat: 11 grams

> **Recipe Tip:** Instead of having a high-glycemic white potato as a side dish that promotes weight gain and energy fluctuations, use steamed or whipped cauliflower. Cauliflower is low on the Glycemic Index and does not promote excess fat storage as does white rice and potatoes.

CURRIED TOFU

Minutes to Prepare: 20

Ingredients

1 cup low-fat extra firm tofu	1 tablespoon raw cane sugar
1 cup 1% milk	1 tablespoon whole wheat flour
1 large onion	2 tablespoons curry powder
1 teaspoon minced garlic	1 teaspoon butter
1 teaspoon minced ginger	1 cup brown rice

Directions

Peel and dice the onion and sauté in a non-stick frying pan with butter until tender. Add milk, garlic, ginger, cane sugar and curry powder. Bring to a boil, while stirring constantly. Mix flour with a bit of cold water and blend completely with a whisk. Slowly add the flour mixture to the curry mixture and cook until a medium thickness is reached. Add tofu cubes and simmer for 10 minutes. Serve over brown or wild rice and enjoy!

Nutritional Facts Per Serving

Total calories: 333
Protein: 23 grams
Carbohydrates: 38 grams
Fat: 11 grams

Recipe Tip: The Glycemic Index rating of instant white rice (69) is significantly higher than that of brown rice (58) or basmati rice (50). Brown rice is loaded with fiber and precious B vitamins. In fact, the processing of brown rice into white rice destroys 67 percent of the vitamin B3, 80 percent of the vitamin B1, 90 percent of the vitamin B6, half of the manganese, half of the phosphorus, 60 percent of the iron, and all of the dietary fiber and essential fatty acids.

BLACK BEAN BBQ CHICKEN WRAPS

Minutes to Prepare: 20

Ingredients

2 8-ounce boneless chicken breasts, cut into strips and cooked

2 whole grain wraps

½ can black beans, drained and rinsed

¼ white onion

½ tomato, diced

1 tablespoon butter

½ cup chopped romaine lettuce

4 tablespoons hickory smoked barbeque sauce

salt and pepper to taste

Directions

Melt butter in a non-stick pan. Add chicken breast strips; cook on medium-high heat for 10 minutes. Add black beans, onion, salt and pepper. Once the mixture is browned, add the barbeque sauce and cook only until the sauce begins to boil. Remove from heat. Spoon mixture evenly down the center of the wraps. Top with diced tomato and lettuce, fold the wraps and serve.

Nutritional Facts Per Serving (1 wrap)

Total calories: 476

Protein: 40 grams

Carbohydrates: 27 grams

Fat: 11 grams

Recipe Tip: Black beans are one of the best sources of cholesterol-lowering fiber. Low on the Glycemic Index and high in iron and magnesium, black beans are a wonderful addition to salads, stews and chili. If beans give you gas, simply soak them overnight.

ZESTY EGG MUFFINS (☺)

Minutes to Prepare: 30 (Eliminate bread if on five-day cleanse.)

Ingredients

3 whole eggs

8 egg whites

½ large white onion

1 cup chopped mushrooms

1 teaspoon butter

1 teaspoon minced garlic

1 tablespoon Tex-Mex seasoning

1 teaspoon salt

½ teaspoon pepper

Directions

Mix whole eggs, egg whites and Tex-Mex seasoning and beat evenly. Set aside in a separate bowl. Melt 1 teaspoon of butter in a nonstick frying pan. Chop onions and mushrooms. Add mixture to pan with garlic, salt and pepper. When mushrooms and onions begin to brown, remove from heat.

Use one large muffin tin with six sections. Distribute onion and mushroom mixture evenly in the bottom. Pour in egg mixture and distribute evenly among the six muffin sections. Bake at 400 degrees for 25 minutes. Remove and serve with a slice of whole grain bread each.

Nutritional Facts Per Serving (3 muffins)

Total calories: 271

Protein: 27 grams

Carbohydrates: 18 grams

Fat: 9 grams

Note: There are many variations of this recipe that can be created simply by changing the ingredients added to the egg mixture. See the next page.

Recipe Tip: Egg muffins can be wrapped with plastic wrap and frozen. Just reheat these great "grabable" protein snacks in the microwave for approximately 2 minutes and enjoy.

GREEK EGG MUFFINS

Ingredients
½ onion
½ cup chopped black olives
¼ cup feta cheese

> **Please note:** All variations below include 3 whole eggs and 8 egg whites.

Directions
Sauté onions and olives in pan. Spoon cooked mixture into bottom of muffin tins. Add egg mixture and sprinkle crumbled feta cheese over top. Bake at 400 degrees for 25 minutes. Remove and serve.

WESTERN EGG MUFFINS (☺) (use vegetarian meat or cheese during five-day cleanse)

Ingredients
½ onion
6 slices of veggie salami or low-fat ham
veggie or low-fat cheddar cheese, shredded

Directions
Sauté onions and salami in pan. Spoon mixture into the bottom of muffin tins. Add shredded cheese to egg mixture and distribute evenly into muffin tins. Bake at 400 degrees for 25 minutes. Remove and serve.

PEPPER MEDLEY EGG MUFFINS (☺)

Ingredients

½ onion
½ red pepper, finely diced
½ green pepper, finely diced

1 small jalapeño pepper, finely diced (This is a hot ingredient so use according to taste.)
½ cup fresh cilantro, washed and finely chopped

Directions
Lightly sauté onion, green and red peppers and jalapeño pepper in a non-stick pan. Add cilantro to egg mixture, mix evenly and distribute into muffin tins. Bake and serve with fresh Mexican salsa (page 267). Bake at 400 degrees for 25 minutes. Remove and serve.

SWEET POTATO SHEPHERD'S PIE (☺) (use veggie cheese if on five day cleanse)

Minutes to Prepare: 45

Ingredients

3 medium sweet potatoes

1 medium white onion, diced

1 500-gram package of ground round veggie meat

1 cup sliced white mushrooms

½ cup veggie or low-fat cheese, shredded

1 teaspoon oregano

salt and pepper to taste·

1 teaspoon crushed garlic

1 tablespoon butter

1 small tin tomato paste (5½ ounces)

Directions

Peel sweet potatoes, wash, dice and steam until tender (approximately 30 minutes). Mash potatoes and place in the bottom of a small baking dish (a meatloaf pan works best). In a non-stick pan, place butter, mushroom and diced onions, and sauté until tender. Add the veggie ground beef, garlic, oregano, salt, pepper and tomato paste. You may want to add ⅛ cup of water to make the mixture creamier. Cook for 10 minutes. Spoon the mixture on the sweet potatoes, top with shredded cheese and bake for 25 minutes at 375 degrees.

Nutritional Facts Per Serving

Total calories: 419

Protein: 32 grams

Carbohydrates: 56 grams

Fat: 8 grams

Recipe Tip: Although this recipe is slightly higher in carbohydrates, it is a much healthier version of traditional shepherd's pie, typically made with ground beef and white potatoes. With delicious sweet potatoes loaded with beta carotene and veggie meat, which is low in calories and saturated fat, this recipe can't be beat!

HEALTHY SLOPPY JOES

Minutes to Prepare: 15

Ingredients

1 500-gram package of veggie ground meat	2 tablespoons Worcestershire sauce
1 14-ounce tin crushed tomatoes	½ teaspoon cayenne pepper (optional)
1 tin tomato paste (5½ ounces)	1 teaspoon butter
1 medium onion	3 tablespoons whole grain flour
1 teaspoon chili powder	2 whole grain Kaiser or hamburger buns
	½ cup low-fat shredded cheese

Directions

Peel and dice onion and cook in butter in a non-stick pan until lightly browned. Stir in the veggie ground meat, crushed tomatoes, tomato paste, chili powder, Worcestershire sauce and cayenne. When the mixture is at the boiling point, sprinkle flour on the mixture and stir to thicken. Toast buns and place on a plate, face up. Distribute the "meat" mixture evenly over the buns and top with low-fat shredded cheese.

Nutritional Facts Per Serving

Total calories: 440
Protein: 36 grams
Carbohydrates: 50 grams
Fat: 11 grams

Recipe Tip: Yum! Who doesn't love the classic Sloppy Joe sandwich? Unfortunately, although delicious, Sloppy Joes are not the healthiest and can exceed 850 calories per meal! By preparing the Healthy Sloppy Joe recipe, you will save on saturated fat and calories, but you will not scrimp on taste. If you have trouble finding whole grain Kaiser or hamburger buns, visit your local health food store.

Snackables

Snacks are an important part of everyone's diet. In fact, for the best weight loss results, I recommend you eat one to two small snacks daily between meals. The following snackable foods are good for you, taste delicious and are an excellent addition to your Natural Makeover Diet.

In order to balance the snacks below and stick to the Pick 3 System of eating, add low-fat cheese or a low-fat yogurt on the side.

The dessert options you will find below are not perfectly balanced. They are however sweeter and healthier options to indulge in occasionally. Enjoy!

HUMMUS (☺)

Minutes to Prepare: 10

Ingredients

1 19-ounce can chickpeas
⅓ cup extra virgin olive oil
1 teaspoon crushed garlic

2 teaspoons cumin
3 tablespoons minced white onion

Directions

Open the chickpeas and drain liquid. Pour into a mixing bowl with olive oil, garlic, cumin and minced white onion. Blend until smooth with a hand blender or in a food processor. Refrigerate and serve with cut-up vegetables such as broccoli, mini carrots, sliced red and green peppers, sliced cucumber or mini tomatoes.

> **Recipe Tip:** If you would like to change the flavor of this dip, substitute 2 tablespoons horseradish or 1 tablespoon curry powder or 1 tablespoon Tex-Mex seasoning for the cumin.

GUACAMOLE

Minutes to Prepare: 10

Ingredients

2 fresh ripe avocados

3 tablespoons diced white onion

juice from ½ fresh lemon

½ red pepper, finely diced

½ teaspoon salt

¼ teaspoon pepper

Directions

Cut avocados in half; remove the pit and scoop out the pulp into a mixing bowl. Finely dice the onion and red pepper and add to the avocados, along with lemon juice, salt and pepper. With a hand masher mash evenly into a paste. Cover and refrigerate. Serve with whole grain bread or cut-up vegetables.

> **Recipe Tip:** In order to avoid your guacamole turning brown, keep the pit of the avocado in the mixture while storing in the fridge.

BLACK BEAN DIP

Minutes to Prepare: 10

Ingredients

1 19-ounce can black beans

3 tablespoons minced white onion

1 teaspoon crushed garlic

2 tablespoons Tex-Mex seasoning

3 tablespoons extra virgin olive oil

½ teaspoon salt

¼ teaspoon pepper

Directions

Open and drain the can of black beans. In a mixing bowl combine beans with onion, garlic, Tex-Mex seasoning, olive oil, salt and pepper. With a hand blender or in a food processor, blend the mixture until smooth. Refrigerate and serve with whole grain pita, whole grain chips or cut-up vegetables.

> **Recipe Tip:** This delicious dip is loaded with filling fiber and ranks very low on the Glycemic Index.

AUTHENTIC TANGY MEXICAN SALSA

Minutes to Prepare: 15

Ingredients

3 whole ripe tomatoes, diced
½ white onion, diced
½ bunch fresh cilantro
1 ripe fresh lemon
1 jalapeño pepper

2 teaspoons minced garlic
3 tablespoons extra virgin olive oil
½ teaspoon salt
¼ teaspoon pepper

Directions

Dice tomatoes and place in a mixing bowl. Finely chop cilantro and jalapeño pepper (very fine), and add to the tomatoes along with the onion, juice of the lemon, garlic, olive oil, salt and pepper. Mix evenly with a spoon. Refrigerate and serve with whole grain pita, whole grain chips or cut-up vegetables.

FANTASTIC FRESH FRUIT DIP

Minutes to Prepare: 10

Ingredients

2 whole bananas
1 whole mango

2 teaspoons cinnamon

Directions

Peel and slice bananas and mango. Place in a mixing bowl with cinnamon and blend with a hand blender or in a food processor. Serve with cut-up fruit such as apples, pears, banana pieces, cherries or strawberries. Add grated dark chocolate for additional flavor and sweetness.

> **Recipe Tip:** It has been shown that 1 to 2 squares of dark chocolate daily is good for your health. Dark chocolate is rich in disease-fighting chemicals called flavonoids, which are beneficial for the heart and arterial blood flow.

SO-GOOD SOY BANANA ICE CREAM

Minutes to Prepare: 90

Ingredients

3 ripe whole bananas

1 cup creamy soy milk

3 tablespoons chocolate syrup

2 teaspoons cinnamon

4 tablespoons chopped walnuts

Directions

Peel and thinly slice bananas and place them evenly on a plate or cookie sheet. Freeze for 30 to 45 minutes. Place 1 cup of soy milk in a plastic container in the freezer and allow to set for 30 minutes.

Remove bananas and soy milk from freezer and place in a mixing bowl. Add cinnamon and blend until smooth with a hand blender or in a food processor. Spoon the mixture into two serving bowls, sprinkle walnut pieces over top and drizzle with chocolate syrup. Serve immediately and enjoy.

> **Recipe Tip:** If you love ice cream but want to stay in your "health groove," this easy dessert is the perfect option. With its creamy texture, sweet taste and walnut crunch, you won't feel like you are missing out on anything!

The Pick-3 System of Eating

Readers have been amazed by the results they've seen using the Pick-3 System of eating … and they're asking for more! Here's the latest information and some essential reminders to help guarantee your natural makeover success.

Hormones and the Pick-3 System of Eating

The Pick-3 System of eating is by far the most effective and long-lasting approach to losing weight, preventing disease and keeping energy up, because it is focused on achieving hormonal balance and proper blood sugar control. Why is hormonal balance so integral to overall health and wellness? Hormones are the most powerful chemical messengers in the body, and they have a cascading effect. In other words, hormones are all interconnected; they are constantly "talking," and they rely on each other. The Pick-3 System of eating teaches you how to eat the right types of carbohydrates, proteins and fats at each and every meal or snack in order to stay hormonally balanced, keep energy up and weight down. As we age, hormonal balance becomes even more critical to maintaining optimal weight and energy, and vibrant, radiant skin.

In order to re-cap the connection between food and hormones, let's examine what happens when you eat a piece of white bread—a refined carbohydrate. When you eat this piece of white bread, it is broken down into glucose (sugar) to be used as fuel for the body. However, due to its high Glycemic Index rating, the refined flour rushes into the bloodstream, and your body responds by oversecreting the hormone insulin to deal with the sugar spike. You now know that an oversecretion of insulin can cause myriad effects such as fatigue, hypoglycemia (low blood sugar), weight gain and mental fogginess. If refined and high Glycemic Index carbohydrates are eaten frequently, blood sugar ratios become out of whack, and this can potentially lead to more serious disease processes, such as Type II diabetes, heart disease, obesity and stroke.

Enter protein. Protein facilitates the release of the hormone glucagon, which breaks down fat and has an opposing effect to insulin. For example, if you eat a piece of white bread your body will secrete insulin. Slap some protein onto the piece of white bread (such as tuna, chicken, red meat or egg whites) and glucagon will also be secreted: this is why adding protein to a meal immediately lowers the secretion of insulin, thereby causing less weight gain. This hormonal yin/yang relationship between insulin and glucagon is also one of the main reasons high-protein diets became so popular. Individuals were eating massive amounts of protein and secreting glucagon, which was breaking down fat. In addition, they were eating very few carbohydrates in order to ward off *any* insulin secretion. I knew people through my practice who were purchasing hamburgers from fast food restaurants and eating the patty, then throwing out the bun in fear of carbohydrates! Although these individuals lost a lot of weight in a short time, they became tired and sick and eventually gained it back. In short, a "completely carb-free life" is not sustainable. This speaks volumes to the fact that the body does NOT want to run on protein. It needs proteins for muscle repair and other bodily functions, but it wants to run on glucose from carbohydrates such as vegetables, fruits, and a small amount of beans and whole grains.

Enter fats. Now that you have read up on all the different types of fats that exist, you can easily decipher between the good and the bad. The good types of fat, such as monounsaturated fats (olive oil, avocados) and essential fats (cold-water fish, sesame seeds, almonds, walnuts, flaxseeds and flaxseed oil), are a critical component of the diet because they too lower the sugar spike and insulin response that can occur when eating too many refined carbohydrates. In addition, these types of fat are necessary for heart health, beautiful skin, brain function, digestion and even for weight loss! Remember, think "sprinkling" when it comes to fat, as it does have more than twice the calories of carbohydrates and proteins!

- Sprinkle nuts onto a salad.
- Sprinkle flaxseeds onto your morning yogurt.
- Put slices of avocado into your sandwich.
- Use olive oil to make your stir-fries.

Now that we have established the necessity and role of the macronutrients—carbohydrates, proteins and fats—and their effect on hormones and blood sugar control, it is important to focus on the types of macronutrients you are eating. The Pick-3 System of eating offers a huge variety of delicious foods that are filled to the brim with nutrients, minerals, precious proteins and essential fats. Simply refer to table 4.3 to discover all the foods you can eat.

Stocking Your Kitchen for the Pick-3 System of Eating

The people I encounter in my professional life often initially come up with a list of excuses as to why they cannot make time for their health. I have heard everything from "I'm too busy!" to "I don't have the energy." In reality, everyone needs to eat and everyone needs to grocery shop. Shopping for healthier foods that will dramatically improve physical and mental health does not take more time. Once you have the information, you are on your way!

Let's face it, when people are stressed, rushed or in the throws of a craving, they tend to turn towards the closest sugary or starchy food such as a muffin or a bagel. Unfortunately, these high GI foods will cause the blood sugar roller coaster discussed above. In other words, they will make you feel worse. In order to easily merge the Pick-3 System into your life, I have found the following tips to be incredibly helpful in stocking your kitchen.

PICK 1—SLOW CARBOHYDRATES

- Keep frozen fruit in your freezer. Options include blueberries, strawberries, mangos, bananas and peaches.

- Purchase sprouted-grain bread and keep it in the fridge or the freezer for a lower-GI grain option. Have you ever noticed breads or wraps that never go bad sitting on your counter? Most organic or sprouted-grain breads do not contain any preservatives and can get moldy quicker than others. Storing them in the fridge or freezer will help them to last longer. As a general rule, one piece of bread should have a minimum of 2 grams of fiber.

- Keep chopped veggies such as cucumbers, carrots, radishes, celery, broccoli, cherry tomatoes and cauliflower in the fridge as a wonderful slow-carbohydrate option to munch on. Cherry tomatoes and red pepper slices are great for cravings.

- Take time to prepare the fresh fruits and vegetables you purchase at the grocery store. Buy healthy dips for your cut-up veggies such as hummus (chickpea dip) or baba ghanoush (eggplant dip).

- Make your plate as colorful as you can by incorporating vibrant-looking fruits and vegetables such as blueberries, tomatoes, broccoli, spinach, carrots and sweet potatoes. The color of fresh produce is one of the best indicators of health. Sadly, one third of all vegetables consumed in the U.S. are iceberg lettuce, French fries and potato chips. It is well documented that people who eat five or more servings of fresh fruits or vegetables per day lower their risk of developing cancer by 50 percent in comparison to those who eat only two servings per day.

PICK 2—LEAN PROTEINS

- Invest in a good protein powder.

- Keep hard-boiled eggs in the fridge. They are a "grabable" protein option that also contains fat. Don't be scared of eggs. They are one of the greatest foods on the planet.

- Have lean meats on hand as easy protein sources.

- Keep yogurt or cottage cheese in your fridge as the ideal snack. Sprinkle with flaxseeds and add berries or bananas for a perfect hormonal balance.

- Try to eat wild Atlantic salmon at least once per week. Most canned salmon is derived from wild sources.

PICK 3—ESSENTIAL FATS

- Stock up on fats that are easily accessible for sprinkling such as almonds, walnuts and sesame seeds.

- Cook with extra virgin olive oil or coconut oil for flavor and stability. Both oils remain stable in chemical structure at medium heat. In other words, you are safe to cook with olive or coconut oil at approximately 350–400 degrees Fahrenheit.

- Avoid nut butters that are loaded with sugar and trans fats. Stick to natural nut butters such as peanut, soy, cashew or almond butter.

- Avoid margarines that are filled with harmful trans fatty acids.

Tips to Following the Pick-3 System of Eating

If weight loss and an increase in energy are your goals, consider the following tips that will help you follow the Pick-3 System of eating:

- If you are going to eat a slow-carbohydrate grain such as whole grain bread or pasta, try to have it at lunchtime. Make your lunch or snack with a grain and make dinner a slightly lighter meal filled with non-starchy vegetables, proteins and a sprinkling of fat.

- Grocery shop and prepare on Sunday evenings. This will ensure you have Pick-3 foods available in your fridge and kitchen such as cut up veggies, fruits, whole grains, natural nut butters, egg whites, lean or soy meats, healthy oils, nuts and seeds.

- Although processed differently by the body, alcohol should be considered a sugary carbohydrate that stimulates insulin. Try to have alcohol with some protein or fat. Whenever possible, try to make your alcohol choice a glass of red wine. Red wine offers a rich source of phytochemicals (plant chemicals) that have been shown to offer protection against various disease processes such as cancer and heart disease.

- Learn to "eyeball" your food and become familiar with Pick-3 serving sizes.

Pick-3 Serving Sizes

The following are average amounts you should eat in a serving:

PICK 1—SLOW CARBOHYDRATES

- 1 serving of fruit (½ cup or 1 small fruit) = 10 grams of carbohydrates
- 1 cup of vegetables = 5 grams of carbohydrates
- ½ cup of beans = 20–25 grams of carbohydrates
- 1 whole wheat tortilla = 12 grams of carbohydrates

- 2 pieces of crisp Wasa bread = 15 grams of carbohydrates
- 1 slice of bread (whole wheat or whole grain) = 15 grams of carbohydrates

Note: It is best to save bagels as an occasional treat as they are very carbohydrate dense, containing anywhere from 25–40 grams of carbohydrates.

PICK 2—PROTEINS

- 1 scoop of protein powder = 25 grams of protein
- 4 ounces of chicken or fish = 28 grams of protein
- 3 ounces of sirloin steak = 25 grams of protein
- ½ cup of egg whites = 13 grams of protein
- 1 ounce of low-fat cheese = 7 grams of protein
- 1 cup of lima beans = 15 grams of protein
- 4 ounces of firm tofu = 10 grams of protein

Note: Try to consume red meat sparingly (i.e., once every two weeks).

PICK 3—"SPRINKLE" FATS

- 1 tsp. of extra virgin olive oil = 5 grams of fat
- 7 almonds = 5 grams of fat
- ⅛ of an avocado = 5 grams of fat
- 1 tablespoon of peanut butter = 5 grams of fat

There will be times—such as weddings, late nights at the office or when you are traveling—that do not permit you to follow the

Pick-3 System of eating. Do not worry. Now that you have the information on how to eat in hormonal balance, you can eat in this manner 80 percent of the time, fall off the health wagon 20 percent of the time, and still reap all the positive results.

references

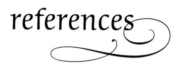

Chapter 2

Brodb, S.A. "Unregulated inflammation shortens human functional longevity." *Inflamm Res.* 2000 Nov; 49(11): 561–70.

Carr, Anitra C., and Frei, Balz. "Toward a new recommended dietary allowance for vitamin C based on antioxidant and health effects in humans." *Am J Clin Nutr.* June 1999; 69: 1086–07.

Collins, David M., and Gibson, Glenn R. "Probiotics, prebiotics, and synbiotics: approaches for modulating the microbial ecology of the gut." *Am J Clin Nutr.* May 1999; 69: 1052–57.

Crook, William G., and Marjorie H. Jones. *The Yeast Connection Cookbook.* Jackson, TN: Professional Books, 1989.

Halliwell, B., et al. "Health promotion by flavonoids, tocopherols, tocotrienols, and other phenols: direct or indirect effects? Antioxidant or not?" *Am J Clin Nutr.* Jan 2005; 81: 268S–76S.

Invitti, C. "Obesity and low-grade systemic inflammation." *Minerva Endocrinol.* Sept 2002; 27(3): 209–14.

Lindahl, B., et al. "Markers of myocardial damage and inflammation in relation to long-term mortality in unstable coronary artery disease. FRISC Study Group. Fragmin during Instability in Coronary Artery Disease." *New Engl J Med.* Oct 19, 2000; 343(16): 1139–47.

Pradhan, A.D., et al. "C-reactive protein, interleukin 6, and risk of developing type 2 diabetes mellitus." *JAMA.* July 18, 2001; 286(3): 327–34.

Sitzer, M., et al. "C-reactive protein and carotid intimal medial thickness in a community population." *J Cardiovasc Risk.* April 2002; 9(2): 97–103.

Ward, P.A. "Cytokines, inflammation, and autoimmune diseases." *Hosp Pract* (Off Ed). May 15, 1995; 30(5): 35–41.

Chapter 4

Connor, W. "Importance of n-3 fatty acids in health and disease." *Am J Clin Nutr.* Jan 2000; 71: 171S–175.

Koh-Banerjee, Pauline, et al. "Changes in whole-grain, bran, and cereal fiber consumption in relation to 8-y weight gain among men." *Am J Clin Nutr.* Nov 2004; 80: 1237–45.

Schanfarber, L. *Alive.* Oct 2004; no. 264: 24.

Simopoulos, A.P. "Omega-3 fatty acids in health and disease and in growth and development." *Am J Clin Nutr.* Sept 1991; 54: 438–63.

Weil, A. *Eating Well for Optimum Health: The Essential Guide to Bringing Health and Pleasure Back to Eating.* Toronto: HarperCollins, 2001.

Chapter 5

Appel, L.J. "Nonpharmacologic therapies that reduce blood pressure: a fresh perspective." *Clin Cardiol.* 1999; 22 (supplement III): III1–III5.

Arnold, L.E., et al. "Potential link between dietary intake of fatty acid and behavior: pilot exploration of serum lipids in attention-deficit hyperactivity disorder." *J Child Adolesc Psychopharmacol.* 1994; 4(3): 171–82.

Belluzzi, A., et al. "Polyunsaturated fatty acids and inflammatory bowel disease." *Am J Clin Nutr.* 2000; 71(supplement): 339S–42S.

Boelsma, E. "Nutritional skin care: health effects of micronutrients and fatty acids." *Am J Clin Nutr.* 2001; 73(5): 853–64.

Bruinsma, K.A., and Taren, D.L. "Dieting, essential fatty acid intake and depression." *Nutr Rev.* 2000; 58(4): 98–108.

de Lorgeril, M, et al. "Mediterranean alpha-linolenic acid-rich diet in secondary prevention of coronary heart disease." Lancet. 1994; 343: 1454–59.

Harper, C.R., and Jacobson, T.A. "The fats of life: the role of omega-3 fatty acids in the prevention of coronary heart disease." *Arch Intern Med.* 2001; 161(18): 2185–92.

Hibbeln, J. "Seafood consumption, the DHA composition of mothers' milk and prevalence of postpartum depression: a cross-national analysis." *J Affect Disord.* 2002; 69: 15–29.

Kremer, J.M. "N-3 fatty acid supplements in rheumatoid arthritis." *Am J Clin Nutr.* 2000; (supplement 1): 349S–51S.

Nordstrom, D.C., et al. "Alpha-linolenic acid in the treatment of rheumatoid arthritis. A double-blind, placebo-controlled and randomized study: flaxseed vs. safflower seed." *Rheumatol Int.* 1995; 14: 231–34.

Okamoto, M., et al. "Effects of dietary supplementation with n-3 fatty acids compared with n-6 fatty acids on bronchial asthma." *Int Med.* 2000; 39(2): 107–11.

Silvers, K.M., and Scott, K.M. "Fish consumption and self-reported physical and mental health status." *Public Health Nutr.* 2002; 5: 427–31.

Simopoulos, A.P. "Essential fatty acids in health and chronic disease." *Am J Clin Nutr.* 1999; 70 (30 Supplement): 560S–69S.

Simopoulos, A.P. "The importance of the ratio of omega-6/omega-3 essential fatty acids." *Biomed Pharmacother.* Oct 2002; 56(8):365–79.

Wensing, A.G., et al. "Effects of dietary n-3 polyunsaturated fatty acids from plant and marine origin on platelet aggregation in healthy elderly subjects." *Br J Nutr.* 1999; 82: 183–91.

WEBSITES

http://www.consumerlab.com/results/omega3.asp

http://www.eggs.ca/nutrition/health/omega3.asp

http://www.fda.gov/bbs/topics/news/2004/NEW01038.html

Chapter 6

Ahmad, Alijada, et al. "Increase in intranuclear nuclear factor B and decrease in inhibitor B in mononuclear cells after a mixed meal: evidence for a proinflammatory effect." *Am J Clin Nutr.* April 2004; 79: 682–90.

Yunsheng, M. "Association between eating patterns and obesity in a free-living US adult population." *Am J Epidemiol.* 2003; 158: 85–92.

WEBSITES

http://www.digestivefacts.com/ms/news/518521/main.html

Chapter 7

Phillips, B., Kato, M., Narkiewicz, K., Choe, I., and Somers, V. "Increases in leptin levels, sympathetic drive, and weight gain in obstructive sleep apnea: heart and circulatory physiology." *Am J Physiology*. July 2000; 279: H234–37.

Scheen, A.J. "Clinical study of the month. Does chronic sleep deprivation predispose to metabolic syndrome?" *Rev Med Lieg*. Nov 1999; 54(11): 898–900.

Spiegel, K., et al. "Impact of sleep debt on metabolic and endocrine function." *Lancet*. Oct 23, 1999; 354(9188): 1435–39.

Spiegel, K, Tasali, E., Penev, P., and Van Cauter, E. "Brief communication: sleep curtailment in healthy young men is associated with decreased leptin levels, elevated ghrelin levels, and increased hunger and appetite." Annals Intern Medicine. 2004; 141: 846–50.

WEBSITES

http://abc.net.au/science/sleep/facts.htm

Chapter 8

Murray, Michael. "Diabetes and hypoglycemia." *Prima Health*. 1994: p. 16.

Nielsen, S.J., and Popkin, B.M. "Patterns and trends in food portion sizes, 1977–98." *JAMA*. Jan 2003; 289(4): 450–53.

Salazar-Martinez, Eduardo, et al. "Coffee consumption and risk for type 2 diabetes mellitus." *Annals Intern Medicine*. Jan 2004; 140: 1–8.

Recipes

http://www.whfoods.com/genpage.php?tname=foodspice&dbid=128